Intermittent Fasting for Women

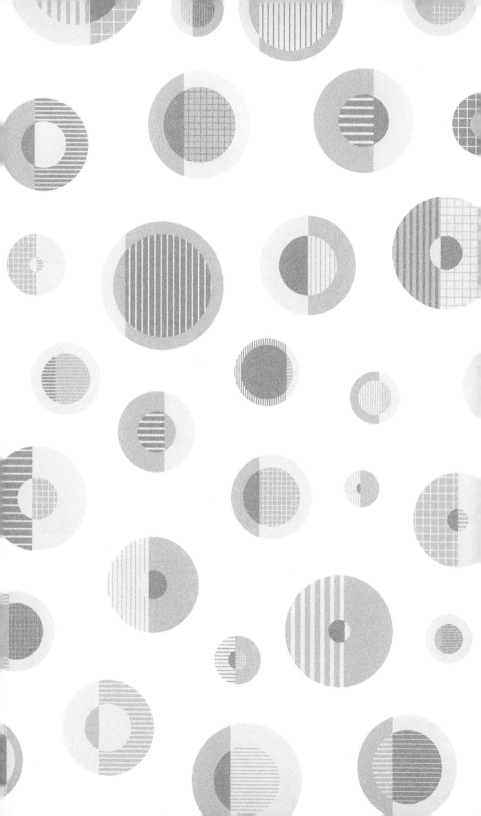

Intermittent Fasting for Women

Guidance and Meal Plans to Reset Your Metabolism and Lose Weight

LORI RUSSELL, MS, RD, CSSD

ROCKRIDGE PRESS

Interior and Cover Designer: Brian Lewis
Art Producer: Hillary Frileck
Editor: Britt Bogan

ISBN: Print 978-1-6461-1164-0 | eBook 978-1-6461-1165-7

R0

This book is dedicated to all those struggling to find an eating style that fits their lifestyle and also promotes good health.

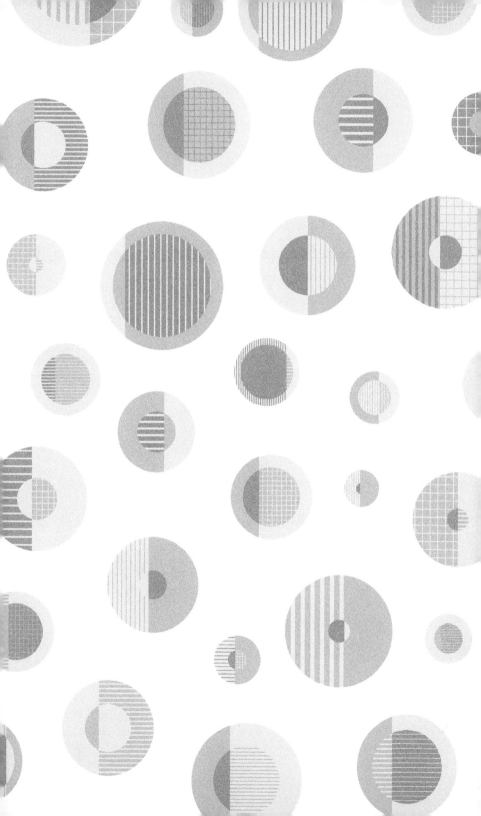

Contents

Introduction

Throughout my twelve-year career as a registered dietitian specializing in nutritional coaching in sports, wellness, and weight loss, I have worked with individuals struggling to have a healthy relationship with food. Part of being able to help people on their healthy-eating journey comes from a deep understanding of how hard it is, and I understand the personal, internal struggle that accompanies each and every food choice. I changed my eating habits from mindlessly munching on junk food to consuming nutritious and thoughtful options that were inspired by my growing nutritional knowledge and expertise. But that didn't necessarily ease the internal struggle of connecting food choices with health and body wellness goals. You likely face stressful questions such as "Should I eat now? Am I *really* hungry? Will this ruin my diet? Should I avoid this? Is this good for me?" several times a day, as diet culture tells us to scrutinize every bite. This same diet culture also leaves us with confusing, mixed messages about losing weight, telling us to restrict what we eat but also eat more frequently throughout the day.

Breaking free of this endless, stressful diet cycle helped me find peace of mind and begin nourishing my body in a stress-free, health-promoting way. Practicing intermittent fasting helped break the diet cycle and allowed me to nourish my body by promoting balance, improving hunger cues, and regulating my hormones.

Let me be clear: Fasting is not starving. It is the prescribed absence of food or drink for a set amount of time. Spending a chunk of my day (mostly while sleeping!) fasting helped take pressure off those nagging "Should I eat this?" feelings because I was simply eating less frequently. Fasting helped improve my body composition by increasing fat metabolism and helped boost my work productivity by allowing my mind to focus less on food choices. In short, the periods of not eating (being in the fasted state) took the strain off the periods of eating (being in the fed state) and ultimately made me a better version of myself, with a healthier body and mind and an improved relationship with food. I'm very excited to share my nutritional expertise and personal experience on fasting throughout this book and hope it will provide you with the benefits that fasting provides.

Don't be fooled by fasting's current popularity in mainstream wellness culture: This is not a fad diet. Far from it. Fasting should be thought of as a lifestyle practice, not as a diet. I'll get into the details of that later, but the practice of fasting is not a new concept. Ancient cultures went without food for a variety of reasons: preparing for battle, attaining religious enlightenment, and engaging in political protest.

This book isn't about fasting's extensive past. It's about fasting's relationship to your health. Numerous health factors are associated with abstaining from calories—improved focus and memory, slowing the aging process, stimulating fat loss, enhancing hormone control, hunger regulation, reducing inflammation, and boosting cardiac output. Because intermittent fasting is flexible and easy to follow, it can be sustained long term as a lifestyle practice. This book is about explaining the various types of fasting practices and how they could stimulate those potential benefits. It's about helping you improve your well-being and exploring fasting's potential to do just that.

Any individual can use fasting periods to improve health outcomes; however, bodies are biologically diverse and those differences affect how fasting can work toward your goals. Generally speaking, women's bodies differ from men's in terms of metabolism, body composition, hormone distribution, reproductive lifespan, temperature regulation, and other basic biological and physiological factors.

Beyond biology, women also face different lifestyle pressures than their male peers. Being responsible for managing a household and providing childcare are examples of this, as is the increased pressure to obtain or maintain a certain physical appearance and stay youthful. These biological factors vary greatly from woman to woman, yes, but they are significant and play a role in how a body and mind responds to adapting to, and succeeding with, a new eating style. Throughout this book, I will explain how fasting can target these biological and lifestyle factors unique to women.

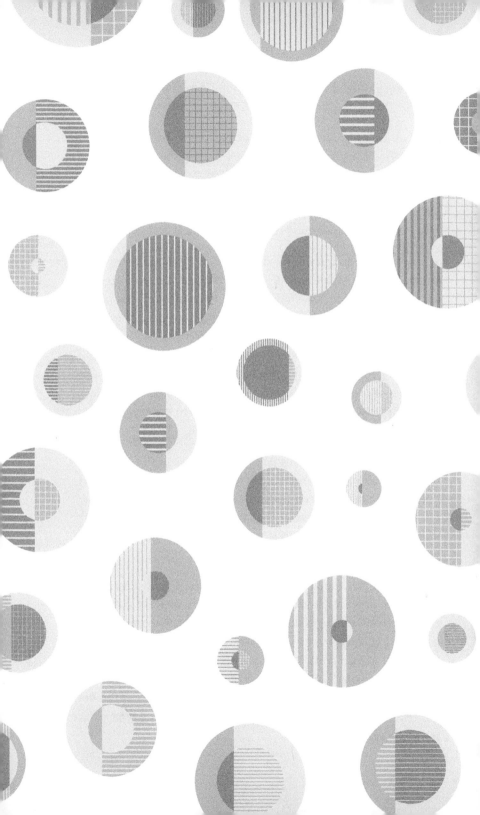

CHAPTER ONE

What Is Fasting?
What Isn't It?

At this point, you are probably bursting with questions about what fasting is and how to do it. This chapter answers those questions. You should leave this chapter feeling more knowledgeable and confident in beginning your fasting journey.

FASTING VS. STARVING

Fasting can seem like a daunting task because the media makes it seem extreme (such as extended hunger strikes or weeklong fasts). Fasting simply means you are going without food for a set time period, which could be as little as 12 hours, and is a natural part of our everyday lifestyle and biological metabolic processes. Unfortunately, fasting and severe calorie restriction tend to get paired together even though they are not synonymous.

Starving is when the body suffers due to a prolonged lack of energy and vital nutrients from food. A person can starve while still eating and drinking; if their food intake is insufficient and doesn't meet their basic daily needs, starvation can occur. Chronic, long-term calorie restriction is a way to starve, deprive, and negatively impact the body.

Fasting is simply a break from food intake—a break that is defined by its duration or intervals, and as part of an otherwise well-balanced eating style that promotes health and energy needs. That is why fasting will not cause any type of serious suffering. Fasting happens naturally for most of us on a daily basis without us even realizing it. Every night while you sleep, you are fasting, unless you happen to wake up for a midnight refrigerator raid. The first meal after you awaken is called "breakfast" for a reason: You are breaking the fast when you consume your morning meal.

THE IMPORTANCE OF HEALTHY FASTING

This book focuses on fasting healthfully and in a way that can help promote and stimulate positive health outcomes. Fasting does this by providing a metabolic reset. Without sounding too buzzwordy, your metabolism can become sluggish over time and require a jump-start to run at full speed again. A sluggish metabolism often limits your potential to reach your health goals. To gain the results desired, such as personal body goals, staying youthful, having efficient digestion, or staying mentally sharp, eating must be approached in a thoughtful, strategic, healthful, and responsible way. I aim to provide you with the information about how fasting can help this process.

I will guide you through popular fasting methods, inform you of how fasting affects a woman's body, the myths surrounding the practice, and the many potential health benefits you may reap from fasting. As you keep reading, learning more, and following the book's advice, it is important you stay true to the guidelines and not attempt to accelerate the process by extending periods of fasting or consuming fewer calories than your body needs. Fasting is, at its core, a way to achieve balance, and balance is not the result of extremes.

SAFETY SIGNALS

Whenever you change your diet, you want to be very aware of how it affects your overall health and be mindful of not risking your safety. Some side effects are bound to occur. Initially experiencing mild to moderate hunger, a little fatigue, and potential moodiness is common as your body adjusts to changes. These symptoms should subside and not seriously affect your health long term. However, your body may reject or resist a new process. If, at any point while fasting, you feel dizzy, faint, nauseated, or experience shaking, migraines, or other indications that you are seriously unwell, it is time to eat. You would be wise to have a nourishing meal and reevaluate what might need adjustment in the future.

MYTHS ABOUT FASTING

When it comes to eating or any popular health topic, real information tends to get obscured by plenty of fake stuff. Let's clarify some of the misconceptions and myths surrounding the topic before moving on to the how-to sections. Here are the most commons questions I've received:

Is fasting unhealthy? Not at all! Short-term fasting is a natural process that most of us experience daily without even noticing.

What is the difference between fasting and intermittent fasting? Technically, all fasting for health reasons is considered intermittent fasting because it is designed to start and stop. This book uses the terms interchangeably.

Isn't not eating food the same as having an eating disorder? No, these are very different things. Eating disorders come from a place of mental control, fear surrounding food choices, and a distorted relationship with how food affects health. Those who fast tend to have a very healthy, positive relationship with food and use the prescribed periods of eating to nourish their bodies thoughtfully.

I've heard that if you don't eat, your body goes into "starvation mode." Is this true? If you eat far less than your body needs for extended periods of time, then yes, your body will work to preserve the stores it has instead of burning them. However, fasting, when done correctly, does not put your body in this compromised position.

Will fasting make my blood sugar drop too low? For most people, fasting works to stabilize and regulate blood sugar levels, allowing your body to have more consistent energy levels.

I want to keep my muscle mass. Will fasting cause my body to eat away at my muscles? Fasting can accelerate fat burning and retain muscle mass. Used in conjunction with a good exercise plan, this process can help you achieve a lean physique.

Won't fasting deprive my body of nutrients? The variety of nourishing foods you'll consume when not fasting is sufficient to sustain your body's needs through fasting periods.

Can't going without food mess up my metabolism? The fact that fasting is intermittent—meaning it starts and stops—helps rev up (not mess up) your metabolism.

If I can't eat, won't I be hangry and cranky? Not eating affects each person's mood differently. If you do experience negative moods, they are likely to pass as your body adjusts to the fast. Also, most of your fast can be done while you're sleeping, if that style works best for you.

I'm worried I'll just binge when I start eating again. Should I be concerned? The process might take a little adjusting to, but fasting should improve and regulate your hunger-satiety levels and cues, allowing your body to eat appropriately for its needs.

I have diabetes. Can I still fast? Fasting can benefit many chronic health conditions by helping to regulate internal factors. If you have a preexisting medical condition, you should consult with a physician before making any lifestyle changes.

I want to keep working out. Isn't that dangerous to do if I'm fasting? You won't have to give up your exercise routine to fast. Fasting workouts can help provide performance adaptations. You'll want to pay attention to your energy levels and adjust the timing of fasting and eating periods to match your workout needs.

Won't fasting mess up my female hormones? When done properly, intermittent fasting can be an effective tool in balancing female hormones. We will touch more on this throughout the book.

THE THREE MAIN METHODS OF FASTING

Now that we've cleared up some common concerns and misconceptions around intermittent fasting, let's dive more into what fasting is. Recall that fasting is the absence of caloric intake for set periods of time. Doing so healthfully requires planning. As a quick introduction to the main styles of fasting for weight loss and health, consider the following:

Time-restricted feeding: In this method, the fasting window spans 10 to 16 hours a day and the remaining hours are non-fasting. During fasting hours, no calories from food or liquid are consumed. Non-caloric substances such as black coffee, water, and plain tea can be enjoyed while fasting. This approach is great for beginners, as a large part of the fasting hours can be spent sleeping and limits the burden of going without fuel. Time-restricted feeding is also known as daily fasting and encompasses the Crescendo and Leangain methods.

Weekly fasting: This is another very popular style that is sometimes referred to as alternate-day fasting and involves a full 24 hours spent fasting or not fasting. Occasionally, these days are lumped together for 48 hours of fasting, but more commonly they alternate throughout the week. The 5:2 approach, where one fasts two days a week and does not fast the other five, is an example of this. On fasting days, individuals consume either no calories or limit intake to a mere 25 percent of daily caloric needs. On non-fasting days, they may resume their typical food intake. Many adopt this style of fasting after starting with time-restricted feeding.

Extended fasting: The most extreme and less common version of fasting, this method involves going a prolonged period before returning to normal food consumption. This kind (a.k.a. "long fasts") involves consuming less than 25 percent of caloric needs for at least 48 hours and up to a full week. This version is more suitable for those with a high level of social support who are seeking to positively shake up their lifestyle or obtain drastic results.

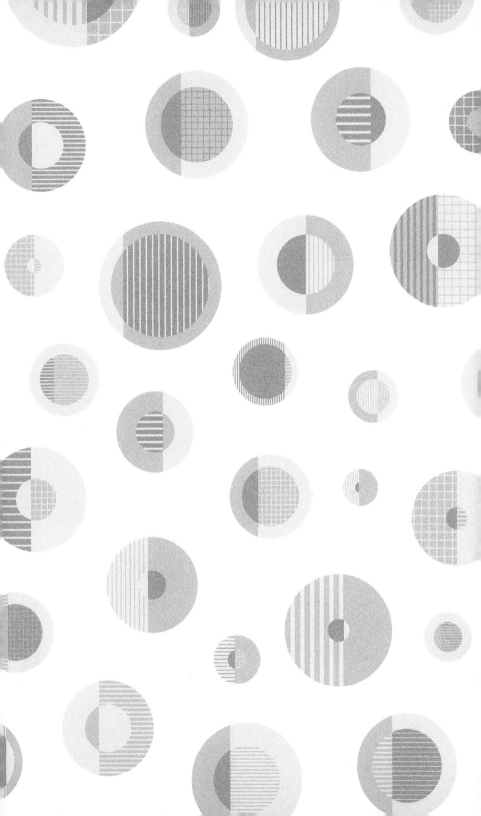

CHAPTER
TWO

Fasting and the Female Body

At this point, I hope you are feeling excited about fasting and have a solid grasp of the fundamentals. While the practice should be easy to conduct (no extra equipment, memberships, or special foods needed), there is still a bit more education to get through before you begin. This chapter covers basic fasting principles and how they uniquely affect and benefit women.

HOW THE TERM "WOMAN" IS USED IN THIS BOOK

Fasting is a practice that can help someone of any gender. However, throughout this text, some specific gender vocabulary will be used. This is not intended to exclude, offend, or alienate anyone, but simply to take a straightforward approach when explaining how fasting uniquely targets the cisgender woman. This text uses "female" and "woman" interchangeably to refer to biological and physiological mechanisms affecting this population, such as reproductive capacities and hormone distribution.

THE NUTRITIONAL NEEDS OF WOMEN

There are many ways fasting and weight-loss recommendations apply to both men and women; however, women have some unique needs, meaning that a few female-specific modifications should be made. Understanding your physiology will help you target your needs and obtain your goals faster. Let's explore several important nutritional needs in more detail so you can feel confident in your approach to better your health throughout this process.

Calcium: While many bodily functions involve this mineral, including heart and nerve regulation, its bone-strengthening aspect is most relevant to women. As we age, estrogen production declines and bone loss accelerates, putting women at greater risk of brittle bones and osteoporosis. To promote your health, rely on whole foods like dairy and leafy greens rather than calcium supplements. Consuming enough vitamin D is also needed to properly absorb calcium in foods.

Magnesium: This mighty mineral is involved in over 600 bodily functions, including enhancing energy metabolism and promoting sleep quality, according to one comprehensive study. Additional research says that it also fights inflammation, high insulin levels, and accelerated aging. Magnesium levels tend to fall throughout the menstrual cycle and should be a focus of any woman's healthful diet.

Folate: According to at least one research study, this mineral directly supports a healthy pregnancy because it prevents neural tube defects in developing infants. Additionally, the Centers for Disease Control recommends all prenatal women, regardless of plans for future pregnancy, get enough of this nutrient. Even if you aren't motivated by reproductive reasons, getting enough folate from sources such as greens, citrus, nuts, seeds, or fortified foods can help your body burn carbohydrates.

Iron: Red blood cells need iron to carry oxygen to tissues and muscles throughout the body. When iron stores become low, the body becomes fatigued due to the inability to transport oxygen. Recommendations say women should take 18 grams a day. This is because you lose iron through menstruation. When you're not fasting, you'll want to focus on consuming iron-rich foods. While many foods contain iron, the body has a very hard time absorbing it from food, and for this reason, a supplement might be worthwhile.

Vitamin C: Your body needs this super vitamin to help absorb more of the iron you eat. Your best bet is to eat it at every meal by consuming healthful fruits and vegetables loaded with this nutrient. Vitamin C also helps skin stay radiant and youthful.

B12: This nutrient plays a large role in energizing your body and revving up your metabolism because of its vital function in processing the macronutrients protein and fat, which can affect achieving your body goals. This nutrient is found in animal products, meaning vegetarians or vegans will need a supplement.

Thiamine: Also known as B1, this compound is essential for carbohydrate metabolism. Consuming enough thiamine will help your metabolism stay high and enable your body to process the foods you consume more efficiently. Foods rich in this vitamin include potatoes, kale, eggs, and many fortified grain products.

While every nutrient—macronutrients, phytonutrients, vitamins, and minerals—is vital to health, paying more attention to those listed here can support your health and metabolism while fasting. During non-fasting periods, consume a balanced, nutrient-rich diet to prevent any deficiencies or fatigue.

METABOLISM AND FAT

Metabolism is a word that sums up how efficiently your body converts food to energy to be used for everything from blinking to working out at the gym. Your basal metabolic rate (BMR) is the amount of energy your body needs to perform basic, involuntary functions such as keeping your heart beating and breathing. Voluntary actions, such as vacuuming or doing a crossword puzzle, create additional energy demands on your BMR, which is known as thermogenesis. The combination of your BMR and thermogenesis is known as your total energy expenditure (TEE), which is the total energy amount needed to sustain and live your best life each and every day.

Metabolism is generally brought up in terms of weight gain or loss when energy balance is out of whack—consuming too much or too little food for the body's energy demands. Note that metabolism is not a static process; it changes constantly based on environment, stress, activity levels, and dietary choices. A slow metabolism can relate to low energy levels and weight gain, whereas an efficient, fast metabolism relates to high energy levels and weight loss. The higher your activity level, the higher your metabolism. There are also select foods and nutrients that specifically work to keep your metabolism high. Your goal is to stay active and fuel that metabolic furnace with nutrients necessary to keep the fire burning. If you stop adding fuel, your energy will stall.

Gender influences metabolic rates, so it helps to know how female physiology can work for or against your body and health goals. Popular media says that women have lower metabolic rates than men. While many publications exaggerate this, an article in the *Journal of Applied Physiology* demonstrates that the basic concept is backed up scientifically and is due to three main factors: body mass, body composition, and hormones.

Body mass: This refers to your overall weight and size, which can promote or depress metabolism; a large body simply requires more energy to stay alive and perform the same activities as a smaller body. Males are typically larger than females, giving men a biologically higher metabolic rate.

Body composition: The composition of that mass also plays a large role in metabolic function because muscle tissue requires more energy than adipose (fat) tissue to maintain.

Hormones: Testosterone promotes higher muscle tissue, while estrogen promotes fat storage. Estrogen specifically promotes the storage of a healthier type of fat called subcutaneous fat that sits away from organs on breasts, glutes, and thighs, and sustains the body's reproductive potential. Men's bodies, even with less fat overall, tend to have a higher distribution of the more dangerous visceral fat that clings around vital organs in the abdominal cavity. The hormones that work to regulate fat, muscle, and metabolic rate for women fluctuate throughout life, which can lead to changes in how you store fat, shifting metabolic levels, and inconsistent dieting results.

These biological differences give men a slight advantage for having a naturally higher metabolism, but that doesn't mean women can't have similar metabolic levels. Fasting can be a great tool for women looking to create a more efficient metabolism without falling into traditional diet culture traps or throwing their hormones out of whack. Past diet culture and weight loss strategies have resorted to drastic tactics—such as grapefruit and cabbage diets or extremely high caffeine doses—to severely limit calorie intake, but failed to provide sustainable, long-term results due to the serious side effects of constant hunger, fatigue, mood swings, and lowered immunity. Depriving the body of energy will slow your metabolic rate and signal your hormones to burn precious muscle tissue and spare fat stores to preserve reproductive abilities. Intermittent fasting, however, does not limit overall energy intake, protects lean tissue, and maintains a higher metabolic rate while accelerating fat burning and regulating hunger signals.

Intermittent fasting creates stability, routine, and consistency within a balanced eating style and works in tandem with the way your metabolism is set up. Since intermittent fasting only requires small windows of not consuming calories and does not necessarily change the type or quantities of food consumed during eating hours, it is a much healthier, more sustainable, and generally easier approach to a lifestyle change that provides better results than fad diets.

THE ROLE OF INSULIN

The pancreas makes insulin, an extremely important hormone that tells your body to either utilize ingested calories immediately or store them for future use. When we ingest dietary carbohydrates, the pancreas releases insulin to control blood sugar levels, preventing them from getting too high (hyperglycemia). When we consume food, specifically carbohydrates, blood sugar levels become elevated. To combat this, our bodies release insulin to reduce, control, and utilize these sugars. However, due to high-stress lifestyles, simple-sugar consumption, and frequent eating, our bodies constantly pump out insulin, making them less sensitive to the intended affects. This insulin resistance leads to a roller-coaster ride of glucose levels, and these spikes contribute to rapid swings in bodily functions and cellular signaling. Energy levels, mood, mental focus, and metabolic functioning are all negatively affected. Overproducing insulin also makes fat loss increasingly difficult since the presence of insulin blocks the body from using stored fat for energy. Controlling insulin levels promotes stable energy levels, reduces mood swings, and improves mental focus because the flow of nutrients and oxygen to cells is enhanced, promoting a faster metabolism and allowing the mobilization of stored fat for energy.

When our bodies become insulin resistant and the healthy function of insulin is lost, we are at risk for diabetes, hypertension, cardiovascular disease, energy swings, moodiness, and stalled fat loss efforts. Specific female reproductive conditions, such as polycystic ovarian syndrome (PCOS), pregnancy, and menopause, can all affect a woman's insulin function. Reproductive hormone fluctuations cause women to crave sweet foods more often than men, which leads to high sugar consumption and a higher potential for insulin resistance. For example, pregnancy changes the way the body responds to and utilizes insulin, and gestational diabetes is a common complication of pregnancy.

Due to the differences in sex hormones and gender distributions of adipose tissue, women tend to have a higher risk of insulin resistance and lower fat-burning capabilities than men, both of which are exacerbated by insulin resistance. During fasting periods, insulin isn't released to regulate carbohydrate metabolism. This break increases insulin sensitivity, restores normal health functions, and allows the body to run on stored fat energy. One study found that blood sugar levels declined by 12 percent and insulin levels decreased by 53 percent over the course of just a month of Ramadan fasting. Promoting insulin sensitivity by having the body rely on fat burning even in the fed state is why many people will take their fasting a step further, pairing it with a low-carb, high-fat (LCHF), or ketogenic diet.

Integral Female Hormones

There are a number of hormones that are integral to a female's well-being when it comes to regulating body functions, composition, and reproductive health.

Estrogen is the main female sex hormone responsible for how the female body develops and functions. It promotes internal sexual maturity, including reproductive function, and external female appearance, including fat storage. When this hormone's level increases or decreases beyond a normal range, the body can suffer a host of complications. While estrogen gets much of the attention, there are many closely intertwined hormones that work together in complex ways to maintain reproductive cycles and general well-being.

Thyroid stimulating hormone (TSH) is secreted by the pituitary gland and stimulates cell metabolism. TSH should be routinely evaluated in women's health physicals and blood panels as it can indicate hyperthyroidism, hypothyroidism, and Hashimoto's disease.

Epinephrine, the fight-or-flight hormone, is a prime example of an adrenal hormone that is easily affected by fatigue and one that can throw the body out of whack, leading to lower energy, inefficient calorie burn, and increased fat storage.

Cortisol is an important hormone that tends to get a lot of negative attention. The adrenal gland produces this steroid hormone that's related to the flight-or-fight response and ramps up stress and inflammation levels. Ideally, we would see elevated cortisol production in the mornings, during exercise, and periods of acute (short-term) stress because it assists with gluconeogenesis, immediate energy for a body in need. After dealing with these situations, the hormone level should decrease. However, cortisol dysfunction happens when levels stay elevated. This happens in response to chronic, constant exposure to stress and consistent high-volume endurance training (think ultra runners). When cortisol stays elevated, normal functioning is negatively affected by some or all of these: increased cravings, insulin resistance, suppression of immune function, rapid aging, interference with the parasympathetic nervous system, digestive issues, storage of excess visceral fat, and elevated risk of heart attacks, and it might even hamper reproductive abilities. The best way to keep cortisol in check is to manage stress. Most of us cannot reduce stress (it isn't feasible to quit your job, take a vacation, forget money woes, etc.), but we can improve the way we deal with our stressors by implementing healthy lifestyle practices such as meditation, therapy, decreased screen time, increased social interaction, and self-care habits. Intermittent fasting can be one of the tools to manage your stress response as it reduces anxiety about traditional diet culture and food choices. It may also work to promote the body's response to acute stress, improving beneficial short-term fluctuations in cortisol levels.

Kisspeptin is a female hormone responsible for cell-to-cell communication, producing other female hormones, and an increased hormonal sensitivity and balance. Each body is extremely individual, and hormones constantly fluctuate; however, the whole system can go haywire by just having one hormone out of your body's normal range. Imbalances happen for many reasons, including lifestyle factors such as poor sleep quality, high stress, inactivity, excessive exercise, smoking, taking certain medications, and food choices.

Nutrient-deficient food and frequent eating contribute to hormone disturbances. Intermittent fasting can calm the system and promote proper hormone function, helping many women regain stability and control over their bodies. For example, short-term fasts such as 12- to 16-hour time-restricted feeding windows can improve TSH's response to natural circadian rhythms and enhance the gallbladder's activation of this hormone. Because the female system is very sensitive to change, anyone currently feeling unbalanced, burned out, or hormonally fatigued is advised to ease into new habits, including fasting, and avoid any abrupt lifestyle changes.

Many women worry that going without calorie intake will further disrupt these hormones, but the opposite is likely true. Fasting is a relatively short-term process and is not designed to starve or malnourish a body. To see the best thyroid and adrenal balancing results, ease into a fasting protocol, starting with short fasting windows that slowly increase over time. To make fasting a successful practice for hormone stability, a well-balanced, nutrient-rich diet with adequate calories, complex carbohydrates, and attention to micronutrients is required. To further assist your hormone function, focus on lifestyle factors outside of diet, such as getting quality sleep, low-intensity exercise, and meditating.

Adrenal Fatigue

Adrenal fatigue is a collection of symptoms thought to occur from demanding, stressful lifestyles that cause the adrenal gland to increase hormone production. While not currently considered a clinical diagnosis, the overwhelming number of women suffering the related symptoms of adrenal fatigue make this condition a cause for concern and a barrier to well-being. Common symptoms include constant fatigue, headaches, sleeplessness, joint pain, brain fogginess, and weight gain.

HOW FASTING WORKS

Healthy diets are typically associated with how much to eat, what foods to eat, and what foods to limit. We are constantly faced with "What should I eat?" Wouldn't it be a relief to spend less mental energy making choices that might promote stress and guilty feelings? In forgoing complicated diets centered around restricting food choices and portions, you can find peace by eating according to the clock. Fasting diets, regardless of the method, are based on periods of time when no calories are consumed. These fasting periods can range from 12 hours to over two days. Before we get into how to choose the fast best for your lifestyle demands and health goals, let's look at the major ways your body beneficially responds to fasting, including acute stress management, improved fat utilization, lean tissue preservation, and increased sensitivity to hunger hormones.

Your body will typically enter a fasted state after 8 to 12 hours, and you will begin to experience fasting's benefits.

First, this time period without food allows the gastric system to fully digest the last meal. Once that meal is completely digested, your stomach can take a food-processing break. This allows blood flow to be directed away from the gut to the brain and muscles to enhance mental focus and physical energy.

Second, not getting food as your body expects forces it to respond to that acute stress. This short-lived stress is actually very beneficial because it requires your body to react and respond, coming back stronger and healthier each time. Chronic stress is different. This harmful, long-term stress happens when the body is overwhelmed and unable to respond to acute stress. According to a 2013 study, enhancing the body's ability to cope with acute stress is part of what promotes physiological benefits of fasting.

As the fasting period continues, you run out of the body's preferred energy source: glucose. As you reach the 10- to 12-hour mark and your body depletes its readily available glucose, it is forced to tap into stored fat for energy production. Using stored fat has many upsides, including that it is a much slower and more intensive metabolic process to use fat for energy than glucose. To better utilize fat during a fasting period, cholesterol production decreases and fat storage is limited by the enzymatic activation. Fat utilization is just one internal benefit of fasting.

At first, this transition might trigger mild headaches, irritability, and fatigue as the body adjusts to utilizing fat for energy and hormones adjust to the body's current state. When food is withheld, ghrelin production is stimulated, causing feelings of increased hunger. In traditional diets, this works against your weight loss attempts because more ghrelin is associated with cravings, increased fat storage, and a decreased ability to maintain willpower. However, in fasting, the cycling of on/off eating periods doesn't excite long-term effects of chronic hunger or starvation. The body quickly adapts to being more sensitive to regulating these appetite hormones according to the fast/fed state. This regulation sensitivity includes secreting human growth hormone (HGH), which ramps up to break down fat for energy and promotes building lean tissue while reducing fat cell accumulation. HGH is suppressed during feeding periods and increased during fasting to preserve lean tissue. One 2003 study showed that HGH levels increase 50 to 2,000 percent during a fast. Women's bodies have been shown to release additional leptin and adiponectin to counteract ghrelin. When the body is fed again, leptin levels increase, signaling that the body is full. When you consistently fast, the on/off cycle improves the signaling of appetite hormones. Basically, consistent fasting helps your body maintain lean tissue and makes fat loss easier because the body becomes more sensitive and better able to respond to fast/fed changes.

Diets that require constant meals and snacks at all hours do not stimulate the same responses and you'll become blunted to what real hunger and satiety feel like, which leads to mindless eating, depressing portion control, and restrictive, unsustainable diets.

When exposed to a prolonged fast, the body begins a tissue rejuvenation process called autophagy, essentially using up old cells and replacing them with newer, healthier ones. Essentially, it is a process of stimulating natural cleansing and detoxing of cells.

Of course, the body is a very complex system and many lifestyle and biological internal factors are at play throughout the fasted and fed periods that vary greatly from person to person. The general synopsis is that fasting might be responsible for improved health outcomes and triggers reactions in the body that do not get stimulated when the body is constantly fed.

THE HEALTH BENEFITS
OF FASTING

Now that you better understand how the body reacts to fasting, let's get to the part you're really here for: the benefits! Many specific health, skin, and mental conditions have been linked to potential positive outcomes with an intermittent fasting regimen. However, you don't need to have a clinical health condition to benefit. Simply wanting to enhance your quality of life, reduce the impact of everyday stresses, be proactive with your health, or improve your body image are reasons enough to try fasting. Whether you want to lose weight, ramp up performance, or reverse diabetes, it is important to talk to a specialist about your goals and develop a fasting regimen specific to you.

Weight Loss

Focusing on diet is a great way to change or manage weight and body composition goals, yet traditional diets are riddled with unsustainable restrictions and ineffectiveness. Fasting, however, focuses on short-term food abstinence, which increases one's ability to stick with the program and creates adaptations of visceral fat loss stimulation and hunger management. A 2016 study found that simply fasting for one full day can mean you take in 30 percent fewer calories for the next three days. This calorie reduction happens naturally due to hormonal signals and a reset metabolism. If fasting for a full 24 hours seems too daunting, fasting for at least 11 hours each day (largely while sleeping) can stimulate weight loss, according to a 2013 study. An overview of fasting and weight loss research shows that most any regimen can induce significant weight loss, with those who have the most weight to lose seeing the largest benefits.

Diabetes Reversal or Management

Aiming to prevent, manage, or even reverse diabetes should be a priority for those diagnosed or at risk. Costly medications, frequent doctor visits, and poor quality of life have individuals seeking a better way to manage this disease, and intermittent fasting could be a valuable part of a lifestyle care plan. Alternating between fasting and fed states has the potential to regulate insulin levels and improve insulin sensitivity. Research in 2014 showed fasting to be a comparable method to traditional calorie restriction in addressing diabetes risk factors such as visceral fat, fasting insulin, and insulin resistance. If you've been dreaming of ditching diabetic medication, you might be in luck. A 2018 case report of diabetic adults put on alternate-day fasting for 10 months saw 100 percent of participants lose weight and reduce most of their medications, all while reporting that the dietary measure was not a huge burden to stick with.

Anti-Aging

There's no denying the pressure put on women to preserve their youth. Preventing the downfalls associated with age and keeping your body looking and feeling in top form is a great way to focus on your well-being for yourself (and not society). A term associated with anti-aging at a cellular level is autophagy. Put simply, autophagy is self-cannibalism, meaning old, fragile, and damaged cells are destroyed and replaced by fresh, new ones. This cellular regeneration promotes longevity and is the key to preventing a host of chronic health issues such as cancer, cardiovascular disease, and neurodegenerative conditions. This is integral to the fasting process because glycogen depletion, which occurs roughly 1 to 16 hours into your fast, ramps up autophagy and promotes longevity and youthfulness through cell rejuvenation.

Cancer Prevention

Cancer is a broad term that includes many variations and severities that stem from genetics (age, gender, ethnicity) and lifestyle habits (smoking, obesity, sun exposure), while other cases simply have no explanation yet. Women have an increased risk of certain cancers, such as breast, lung, thyroid, and uterine. Think of a good diet as preventive care. Intermittent fasting can be a way to defy your odds of developing cancer. Since traditional calorie restriction is not sustainable, intermittent fasting is a way to get the benefits without the struggle and deprivation. Most of the inherent benefits appear to stem from the aforementioned ability of autophagy to kill off damaged cells and replace them with healthier cells, thus reducing the risk of cancer and allowing the body to fight off or replace potential cancerous cells.

Alzheimer's Prevention

Degenerative mental conditions, such as Alzheimer's, Parkinson's, and dementia, are devastating conditions. They are largely caused by genetics, but high-stress lifestyles may also contribute. Intermittent fasting might be a tool to combat stress's harmful impact on our brains. There are certain bodily processes that only happen in the absence of food. Typically, your brain runs on glucose for energy, but when the body has used up its stores of liver glycogen during a fast, it switches over to relying on fat for fuel. Using fat produces ketone bodies, which are thought to promote quicker synapses and stronger neurons. Think of fasting as a mental challenge; your brain should still be able to function sharply when there is no immediate source of food, and fasting stimulates this process.

Heart Health

Cardiovascular health refers to the health of your heart, veins, and blood. Much of what positively promotes heart health is how your body metabolizes fats and sugars. Diets high in unhealthy fats and refined sugars can promote plaque and cholesterol buildup. Because of this, it is very important to maintain a high-quality diet during the feeding periods of your fasting routine. A review of current research indicates that short-term fasting can have a positive impact on cardiovascular health. These beneficial effects include lower blood pressure, decreased fat surrounding organs, and an improved lipid profile.

Chronic Inflammation Decrease

Inflammation is likely the biggest negative influence on all poor health conditions, whether physical or mental. Acute inflammation is a positive thing, as it essentially tells the body there is an issue that requires immediate attention. This triggers cells to jump into action, rebuild, and repair. Think of it like going out for a run—the exercise makes your muscles sore, but because of that exercise, your cells rebuild and come back stronger. Without that activity and soreness, there is no opportunity to become stronger. The problem comes when that inflammation does not dissipate due to constant exposure to physical and mental stressors such as money, drama, kids, work deadlines, pollution, chemicals, and over-processed foods. While we cannot rid our lives of stress, we can help the body react more positively to that stress. Intermittent fasting has been shown to reduce C-reactive protein and cytokines, internal markers of stress. Giving your body a break from constantly consuming food allows it to target and care for areas outside the digestive system.

Other Areas That Can Benefit from Fasting

You do not have to be currently suffering from (or even concerned with the potential of someday suffering from) a chronic health condition to benefit from fasting. In addition to chronic conditions, there are many other areas of health and bodily functions playing a role in our overall, daily well-being that can be positively influenced by intermittent fasting.

Rheumatoid Arthritis

Rheumatoid arthritis is a crippling condition involving highly inflamed joints that make simple, daily tasks extremely painful and difficult. Since intermittent fasting has been shown to reduce inflammatory markers, it is hypothesized that it would help treat this autoimmune disorder.

Asthma

While there's not yet conclusive data that dietary measures can cure or prevent asthma, current information suggests that calorie intake breaks can reduce flareups. This is thought to be due to the acute stress and regeneration of immune cells.

Skin Conditions Such as Psoriasis and Eczema

Skin conditions can be easily visible and may impact your emotional and mental health. Fasting has been shown to decrease chronic inflammation, so there is high potential for autoimmune-based skin conditions, such as psoriasis and eczema, to be similarly reduced. Since non-caloric beverages are allowed during your fast, you will likely be well hydrated, which improves skin health.

Athletic Performance

Whether you work out now and then or are a well-trained athlete, I am sure you've debated whether or not to eat before a morning workout. Training in the fasted state allows the body to tap into fat for fuel, which is a longer-lasting, slower-burning energy source. Other performance-enhancing adaptations include better muscular and mitochondrial adaptations and improved glucose sensitivity, especially in endurance athletes. It is important to remember that energy levels will be compromised during fasted workout sessions, so intense training is not advised, and even lower-intensity training might feel more difficult than exertion during the fed state. Not to worry though; the adaptations will still be happening and allow for better output when you decide to return to fed training.

Improved Gut Health

Physicians and nutrition experts agree that gut health is an important indicator of overall well-being. Unfortunately, many women suffer from gastric distress such as bloating, IBS (irritable bowel syndrome), flatulence, and sluggish digestion. The typical diet structure of consuming frequent meals puts a high amount of stress on the gastric system to constantly process food. Taking a break from consuming meals and snacks allows the GI tract to fully digest, process nutrients effectively, and have a period of rest. If you experience gastric issues, fasting might ease your distress.

It is important to remember that although the research on how all these health conditions are affected by fasting is promising, more women-focused research is needed to account for the wide variety of health factors and intermittent fasting styles. These conditions are also extremely individual and your specific health status, type of fast you try, how well you nurture your body when not fasting, and other lifestyle factors can greatly affect your personal outcomes. I suggest getting a full physical and blood tests from your physician before undergoing a fast in order to effectively monitor the changes in biomarkers such as insulin, body fat, cholesterol, blood pressure, vitamins, and minerals.

WHO SHOULD NOT FAST?

Fasting is an eating style that most people can greatly benefit from. However, there are always exceptions and fasting might not be the best or safest technique for everyone; a selection of those individuals is listed below. There are individuals who will not respond well to, or should not even begin, a fasting regimen. Fasting for your health requires a great deal of self-awareness, patience, and paying attention to your personal body cues. Feeling some hunger, fatigue, and moodiness in the first few days is very normal as your body adjusts hormones and sensations accordingly, but being able to know this mild discomfort from putting your body in a place of feeling unwell is key to reaping benefits without harm. Throughout your fast, listen to your body and if you become faint, shaky, or dizzy, or suffer any major health concern, it is time to abandon the fasting protocol and reevaluate. It is always a good idea to enlist the support of a physician and dietitian before or during your fast, especially if you have an underlying chronic health condition.

Individuals who may not benefit from fasting include:

Anyone struggling with or prone to an eating disorder: This is a gray area and very individualistic. Following a fasting protocol is not meant to limit food intake and, therefore, might be a way to help people control their eating without actually restricting it. However, those with disordered eating tendencies might feel triggered to push the limits of what the fast is intended for, negating any potential benefits and likely creating a harmful situation. Those currently struggling with an eating disorder should seek treatment for that before ever considering a fasting regimen.

Anyone who is malnourished: Fasting should improve your health, but it might not be right for gaining weight or replenishing nutrients. Those who are currently clinically underweight or depleted of nutritional markers should work to correct those issues first.

Anyone under 18 years old: Children and teenagers have greater nutritional and caloric needs to meet physical and mental growth demands and the energy expenditures of active youths. This population should not be put on an eating protocol that limits access to meeting those needs, as this could lead to malnourishment and form an unhealthy relationship with food later in life.

Pregnant women: Supplying nutrients and energy to a growing baby while maintaining the mother's own health requires frequent fueling. During this time, a woman should pay attention to fully nurturing herself and her baby's needs without feeling confined to any eating-style protocol.

Breastfeeding women: Women breastfeeding after pregnancy should delay fasting until they are finished breastfeeding since it requires attention and awareness to the mother-baby bonding process. Frequent eating to supply additional calories and nutrients is needed for milk production. A fasting regimen can be started once breastfeeding has ceased and the mother is feeling stable and healthy.

Athletes: An athlete's energy expenditures are vastly different depending on the sport. A golfer has a very different energy requirement than a marathon runner. Most athletes will benefit from at least one style of fasting, but those experiencing extreme energy expenditures, who are at risk for nutritional deficiencies, or who are training at multiple intervals throughout the day will likely not benefit from fasting.

Anyone taking daily medications that require consumption with food: See "Medicine and Fasting" sidebar.

MEDICINE AND FASTING

Medications alter how the body responds to different stressors and diet applications in order to provide their intended benefits. Many medications (such as common aspirin) should be taken with food or drink, which slows or enhances absorption into the bloodstream. To ensure your medication is being properly absorbed, the timing of taking these meds might need to be adjusted to fit within your fed windows. The label should indicate whether or not your medication is to be taken with or without food. Most medications will not present any ill effects as long as the fast is done intermittently, extended fasting periods are avoided, and the diet is adequate and healthful during the fed periods. However, there are a few drug classes that may present adverse side effects during a fast. These include immunosuppressants, antidepressants, antibiotics, retro-antivirals, insulin, and angina medications. Taking medications for diabetes might exacerbate the insulin-lowering effects fasting should provide, causing a risk of hypoglycemia. Additionally, many medications (Adderall, for example) are known to alter appetite and might not be appropriate in combination with restrictive dietary measures. Create a list of your current medications and the doses, when you take them, and what you take them with to get a better idea of how your regimen might change based on the type of fast you want to try, and then consult your physician or pharmacist before adjusting the timing of medications or making any drastic dietary changes, including fasting.

HOW TO CHOOSE WHICH METHOD WORKS BEST FOR YOU

Fasting is a blanket term describing any eating style that involves prescribed, scheduled periods of not consuming calories followed by normal food and drink consumption. As I mentioned earlier, fasting for health is a bit more involved than simply eating and not eating. Instead of arbitrary, non-specific periods of not eating, think about your fast as a plan of action that targets your individual health or weight goals. You want to pick the fasting style that best fits your lifestyle and goals so that it feels easy to adapt, setting you up to successfully achieve your desired results. This will increase your level of drive, focus, and commitment to stick with the change.

We covered the main types of fasting in chapter 1. Now we'll apply those styles and discuss which one might best suit your lifestyle and desired outcomes. In chapter 3, we'll cover how to integrate fasting into your lifestyle. It is important to have a good grasp of what your goals, support system, and daily schedule entails. Take a moment to jot down the details of your desired fasting outcomes. Are you looking to just experiment and see what happens? Or are you trying to lose body fat or target a specific health condition? Additionally, list your daily requirements, including things like when you typically wake up, go to bed, eat meals, exercise, work, etc. These details will help you determine the most appropriate fasting style so that your lifestyle isn't significantly or negatively affected.

Intermittent fasting, a style that focuses on time-restricted eating, is a great way to ease into fasting, starting with eight hours and eventually getting to 12 to 16 hours of fasting. The eating window can be adjusted depending on your lifestyle and daily activities. Morning people who are up early and active right away will benefit more from an eating window that begins and ends earlier, such as 9 a.m. to 6 p.m. Night owls can eat from 2 p.m. to 10 p.m. to keep productivity going late into the evening. This flexible style helps those who want to focus on restricting time, not food, which can be a helpful mental trick to stick to fasting.

A 2014 study demonstrated that time-restricted eating has been helpful for improving cardiac health, gaining lean tissue, losing weight, improving sleep, increasing energy levels, and reducing cancer incidences.

Alternate-day fasting requires a little more commitment but is ideal for planners. Those who enjoy meal planning, have long days (early wake ups to late evening commitments), or have set work/life schedules are likely to succeed with this kind of fast. This style can incorporate one, two (as is popularized with the 5:2 style), or even three fasting days a week. Reducing intake like this has been associated with significantly improving diabetic outcomes and insulin sensitivity. It might also be the best plan for those looking for improved mental focus, inflammation reduction, and resolving digestive issues.

Only those with previous fasting experience and the ability to plan their eating schedules for a month or more should participate in extended fasts that last two days or more. Long-term fasts come with the most potential for adverse side effects because energy is severely restricted for 48 hours or more. However, if managed well, this might provide very effective changes in autophagy, benefiting physical and mental aging.

Factors to Consider When Choosing a Fasting Style

Our bodies are naturally set up to work within a set rhythm through a network of complex internal interactions. These interactions get influenced, for better or worse, over time by how we choose to live our lives. Intermittent fasting helps restore our rhythms in a way that supports health and energy.

The circadian rhythm: Your circadian rhythm is your body's 24-hour biological cycle and includes sleeping, waking, energy production, and hunger levels affecting your behavior, energy, and metabolism. External cues such as sunlight, temperature, and food intake all influence this rhythm. Disruptions such as night shifts, screen time, and irregular eating times can impact this natural cycle, causing restlessness, anxiety, insomnia, and excessive cravings. Research from 2016 indicates that poorly timed meals, such as eating late-evening meals when melatonin levels are high, and frequent meal consumption can lead to a dysfunctional metabolism and disrupted biological rhythms. Fasting helps control meal timing and can therefore help restore your body's sleep-wake cycle.

Ghrelin and leptin: The hormones ghrelin and leptin travel between the gut and brain to control and regulate feelings of satiation and hunger. Leptin is stored in fat cells; the more fat cells you acquire, the more leptin the body makes. This hormone signals that you are satisfied, do not need food, and should pull energy from stored fat. On the flip side, ghrelin stimulates appetite. Ideally, these hormones work together to regulate when you do and do not need energy calories. However, like all hormones, your body can become resistant to these signals, throwing everything out of whack. Stress, chronic inflammation, excess body fat, eating several meals a day, and inconsistently consuming meals can all contribute to an imbalance of ghrelin and leptin—largely responsible for food cravings and weight gain. Research has shown that ghrelin levels rise when fasting, but only immediately, stabilizing again after just 1 to 2 days. This explains why you may feel hungrier when initially starting a fast. Luckily, women experience a boost in leptin during a fast. This counteracts the hunger-stimulating ghrelin, returns hormones to normal levels, and prevents you from feeling hungry. It also helps stimulate fat burning as the fast continues long term. Fasting essentially works to reset and stabilize these gut hormones by limiting the frequency of meals, allowing the body to fully digest food, and providing time needed to send, receive, and react to hormonal signals properly.

Eating at night: For those hesitant, overwhelmed, or intimidated by the thought of intermittent fasting, the best and easiest first step you can make is simply not eating at night. This is one of the initial problem areas I address when working with a new client on their nutrition care. Eating at night, when we are less active, means the food is more likely to be stored as fat. However, feeding your body when activity levels are peaking, like late morning through early evening, promotes an active metabolism. Of course, there are individuals who are very active late into the night and require a different fueling schedule, but the majority of us tend to be less active then and need less fuel.

Besides taking in calories when we are not burning them, the foods we choose at night tend to be less nutritious than the foods chosen in the morning. Common night snacks are ice cream, chips, and alcohol—foods that flood the system with sugars and fats. Snacks picked in the afternoon are more likely to be an apple, hard-boiled egg, or hummus with vegetables—foods that provide fiber and nutrients. Sleep is very important to weight loss, and eating close to bedtime messes with your natural circadian rhythm, throwing off melatonin production, altering the production of ghrelin and leptin, and lowering overall sleep quality.

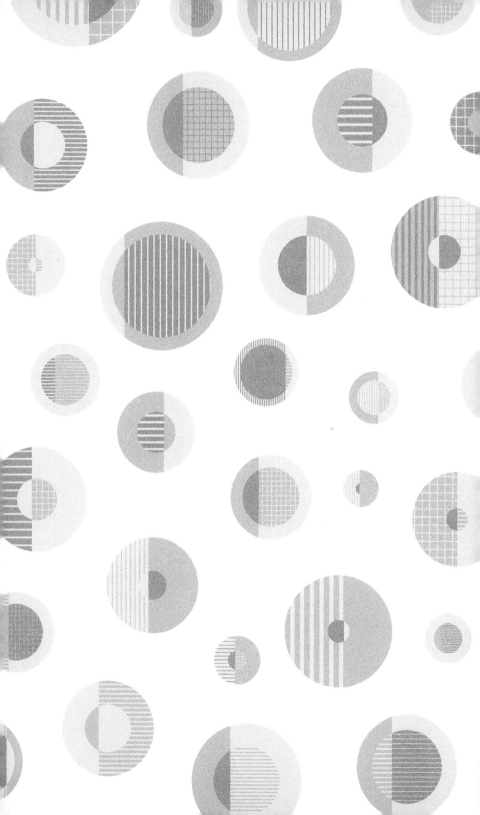

CHAPTER THREE

The Meal Plans

Traditional diet styles fail largely because they are too restrictive, burdensome, or impractical to stick with long term. No one will be successful feeling deprived all the time. Intermittent fasting takes a different approach. Instead of obsessing and fretting over "bad" foods, "good" foods, and portion sizes, you focus on the pattern and routine of your fast and fed periods because there are no food lists or off-limit ingredients, just off-limit times.

This creates stability and allows for plenty of flexibility, making intermittent fasting an excellent approach for improving lifestyle behaviors and long-term success. Ideally, you nourish your body with nutritious, well-balanced food options during the fed periods. To get the best results, define your goals and desired health outcomes, create a way to ease into the full regimen, and consult with a physician and dietitian before starting your intermittent fasting plan.

FASTING PLANS

The concept of fasting is relatively straightforward but implementing any new routine can be intimidating. The following plans will familiarize you with the two primary styles of fasting (daily and weekly) and guide you through choosing one. These plans are designed to provide an example of how to conduct your fasts; you can always switch between plans to find the one that fits your lifestyle best. When not fasting, nourish your body with the highest quality ingredients you are able to obtain from healthy, satisfying fats, muscle-building plant and animal proteins, whole fiber-rich grains, and a plethora of antioxidant-rich fruits and vegetables.

DAILY FASTING PLANS

Intermittent fasting that restricts fed and fast periods to a daily basis is often called time-restricted feeding (TRF). There are several different TRF plans: 12/12, 14/10, 16/8, and 20/4. The numbers indicate how much of 24 hours will be spent fasting and fed. Most women should begin with the 12/12 style, which allows the body to ease into fasting with equal fasting/fed windows and greater flexibility. This 12/12 style is sometimes referred to as the Crescendo method. Some will find this approach suitable and beneficial with no need to increase fasting periods, while others will choose to progress to the 14/10 or 16/8. These longer TRF styles are commonly referred to as the Leangains. The 20/4 style is more extreme and is sometimes referred to as the Warrior method. The following plans provide a guideline for how to approach these different daily fasting styles. The style you choose should fit your life without too much interference. It is also completely fine to rotate between different TRF plans. For example, you might enjoy the 12/12 style six days a week with one day strictly confined to 20/4.

With these daily styles of intermittent fasting, no source of calories should be consumed during your fasting time. This means no food or drink whatsoever outside of black coffee, water, and unsweetened teas. Once fasting is complete, it is time to nourish your body with calories from whole, nutrient-rich foods. Many people opt to skip breakfast or dinner due to the shorter eating window, but this is not always required. The number of meals and snacks you eat depends on your chosen time frame. With longer feeding windows, you can consume meals and snacks on a relatively normal schedule. With shorter feeding windows, you will choose less frequent meals and snacks.

Daily intermittent fasting's biggest benefit is the ease in adapting to the process because of its flexibility. For those not ready to make big food changes, there is also no pressure to regulate, track, or obsess over choices. Simply stick with your time schedule and let the rest fall into place as your body and metabolism responds. To maintain eating by the clock, aim to consume relatively similar meals each day, with meal prep once or twice a week. With any lifestyle change, there might be an adjustment period where you feel stressed about the timing or hungry and irritable from waiting to eat. These minor side effects should subside after the first week. Instead of focusing on the fact that you can't eat, focus on being productive or improving your life in other ways, such as practicing meditation, yoga, reading, or getting chores done. You might be amazed by all the positive things you accomplish when not snacking all evening! A downfall of TRF is that it requires an ongoing, daily commitment of scheduling your food intake by the clock. However, to ease that issue a bit, research shows that doing this even five days a week (free weekends) is beneficial.

12/12-Hour Fast Every Day (a.k.a. Crescendo)

For women unsure of where to begin, the Crescendo method, or 12/12 plan, is a great place to start and is best for those who need a lot of flexibility, because you can eat from 7 a.m. to 7 p.m. one day and 10 a.m. to 10 p.m. the next. As long as the periods between eating last at least 12 hours, you are doing it right. Freelancers, women with young children, and athletes might be more compatible with this fasting approach. Women who are currently feeling burned out or run down or dealing with hormonal imbalances are advised to slowly work their way into the full 12 hours. Instead of going all-in tomorrow, take a few weeks to ease into it. For example, this week, simply track when you naturally stop eating (snacks, alcohol, etc.) and when you reach for your first bite in the morning. The next week, commit to fasting for eight hours every day of the week. This should be simple because you will mostly be sleeping during the fast. For the third week, extend your fast to 10 hours, and finally get to 12 hours after a month of easing into the process. Letting your body slowly adjust to fasting will help you understand which time schedule works best for you, keep you from feeling overwhelmed, and will allow your body's hormones and metabolic processes to adapt.

On this plan, it is important to define your fasting windows in order to be accountable and committed. As I mentioned earlier, they come with a lot of flexibility, but you still have to define them. Think about your daily work schedule and exercise times and how they will be impacted by your choice. Most women will find success consuming calories earlier in the day, as their bodies burn fat slowly and tend to have finicky digestive systems compared to males. Women also tend to crave more sweets, which leads to overeating in the evening. Ending the eating window several hours before going to bed will help improve digestion, promote an efficient metabolism, and prevent snacking on unneeded sweets at a time they're more likely to be stored as fat. This plan should help you tune in to your hunger levels, circadian rhythm, and work to naturally reset and refine habits.

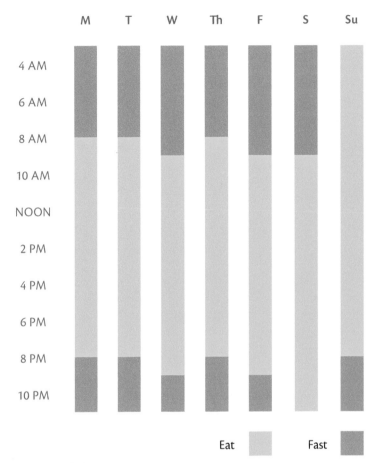

	M	T	W	Th	F	S	Su

Eat ⬜ Fast ⬛

12/12 Meal Plan

Here is a sample plan to follow once you have eased into your time-restricted feeding schedule. This plan is for five days a week of a 12-hour fast and 12-hour eating window, the easiest method shown to have benefits associated with intermittent fasting and an excellent starting point for anyone interested in the lifestyle change. You can generally eat three full meals and even have a snack if you need it. This sample also includes a few time variations to show how flexible it is.

MONDAY (FAST 8 P.M.–8 A.M.)

- 8 a.m.: Breakfast (Break the fast!) – Two pasture-raised eggs with sprouted whole-grain toast, avocado, and cut fruit
- 1 p.m.: Lunch – Bowl of baked tofu, quinoa, spinach, tomato, and roasted red peppers topped with walnuts and drizzled with olive oil and lemon, served with an apple
- 7 p.m.: Dinner (Remember, the goal is to completely finish eating by 8 p.m.) – Chipotle grass-fed flank steak with grilled onions, zucchini, and potatoes; piece of dark chocolate

TUESDAY (FAST 8 P.M.–8 A.M.)

- 8 a.m.: Breakfast – Two pasture-raised eggs with sprouted whole-grain toast, avocado, and Greek yogurt
- 1 p.m.: Lunch – Bowl of free-range grilled chicken, quinoa, spinach, tomato, and roasted red peppers topped with walnuts and drizzled with olive oil and lemon, served with an apple
- 7 p.m.: Dinner – Shrimp tacos in corn tortillas with leftover grilled veggies and fresh salsa

WEDNESDAY (FAST 9 P.M.–9 A.M.)

- 8 a.m.: Breakfast – Greek yogurt with nut butter, muesli, and fruit
- 1 p.m.: Lunch – Free-range chicken Cobb salad with balsamic vinaigrette
- 3 p.m.: Snack – Apple and piece of dark chocolate
- 8 p.m.: Dinner (Extending your eating window leads to extending the fast to 9 a.m. the next day) – Whole-grain pasta with vegetables and tomato sauce

THURSDAY (FAST 8 P.M.–8 A.M.)

- 9 a.m.: Breakfast (At least 12 hours after eating the night before) – Greek yogurt with nut butter, muesli, and fruit
- 1 p.m.: Lunch – Kale salad with tahini dressing and spicy chickpeas served with an apple
- 7 p.m.: Dinner (Eating early means you can break the fast earlier the next day) – Wild salmon roasted in ghee with broccoli and mushrooms

FRIDAY (FAST 9 P.M.–9 A.M.)

- 8 a.m.: Breakfast – Two pasture-raised eggs with sprouted whole-grain toast, avocado, and cut fruit
- 1 p.m.: Lunch – Chicken Cobb salad with balsamic vinaigrette
- 3 p.m.: Snack – Apple with almond butter
- 8 p.m.: Dinner (You can stop worrying about timing until Sunday night) – Grass-fed burger with sweet potato fries and a glass of wine

SATURDAY (NO RESTRICTION)

- 9 a.m. – Break your fast with a balanced meal.
- Eat throughout the day and evening as desired, paying attention to hunger cues and making healthful choices, but also enjoying your freedom!

SUNDAY (NO RESTRICTION–8 P.M.)

- Eat throughout the day without time restrictions.
- Try to put some time aside to prepare meals for the rest of the week to make the process easier.
- Stop eating by 8 p.m.

14/10 and 16/8 (a.k.a. Leangains)

This daily fasting style is a slightly more restrictive version of the Crescendo method. This style might be the best way to accelerate fat burning. By extending periods of fasting, you further tap into your body's ability to pull from stored energy. While it is more restrictive, the 8 to 10 hours of eating still allows for plenty of time to consume nutrient-rich meals and doesn't deprive the body at all. Most women will find it easiest to fast a couple hours before bed and well into the morning. Of course, this can be tailored to work on your own individual schedule. Beyond the longer fasting window, there is less flexibility with this style. Consistent feeding times work to keep hormones, glucose, and hunger from getting out of whack.

This generally works great for women who have been doing well on the Crescendo method and are looking to try a more fine-tuned approach. This tighter feeding period is ideal for those who have set daily routines. Whether you get too caught up in work to worry about a meal, generally dislike having to shop/cook/prepare food, or just would feel better and less stressed making fewer food choices, this is a great plan to help take the pressure off. It might be more difficult for athletes with full-time careers to follow because the eating window would have to be very carefully timed around physical activity to ensure the body has the correct nutrients to thrive and perform optimally.

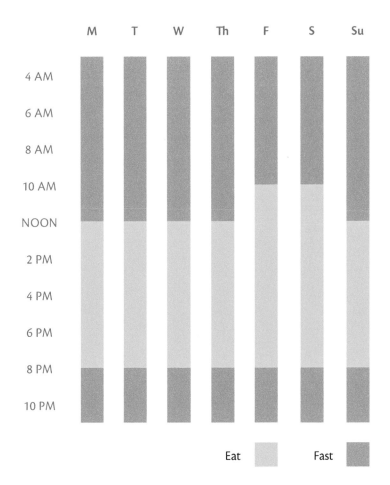

	M	T	W	Th	F	S	Su
4 AM							
6 AM							
8 AM							
10 AM							
NOON							
2 PM							
4 PM							
6 PM							
8 PM							
10 PM							

Eat   Fast

14/10 and 16/8 Meal Plan

Here is a sample plan to follow once you have eased into your time-restricted feeding schedule. This example follows a set time schedule of 16/8, with weekends on the more relaxed 14/10 to show how you can adopt the style while still maintaining flexibility and not giving up your weekend fun.

MONDAY (FAST 8 P.M.–NOON)

- Noon: Lunch – Vegetable omelet with potato hash and fruit
- 4 p.m.: Snack – Nut and date–style energy bar
- 7 p.m.: Dinner (Remember, the goal is to completely finish eating by 8 p.m.) – Miso butter grass-fed flank steak with sautéed tomatoes and zucchini; piece of dark chocolate

TUESDAY (FAST 8 P.M.–NOON)

- Noon: Lunch – Grilled chicken and vegetable wrap served with a yogurt
- 4 p.m.: Snack – Two hard-boiled eggs and an apple
- 7 p.m.: Dinner – Lentil Bolognese pasta

WEDNESDAY (FAST 8 P.M.–NOON)

- Noon: Lunch – Chicken Cobb salad with balsamic vinaigrette
- 4 p.m.: Snack – Nut and date–style energy bar
- 7 p.m.: Dinner – Wild salmon with balsamic roasted beets, arugula, and brown rice

THURSDAY (FAST 8 P.M.–NOON)

- Noon: Lunch – Vegetable omelet with potato hash and fruit
- 4 p.m.: Snack – Apple with almond butter
- 7 p.m.: Dinner – Baked falafel with cucumber, tomato, and tzatziki salad

FRIDAY (FAST 8 P.M.–10 A.M.)

- Noon: Lunch – Greek yogurt with muesli, nuts, and fruit
- 4 p.m.: Snack – Cut vegetables and hummus
- 7 p.m.: Dinner – Grass-fed burger with sweet potato fries

SATURDAY (FAST 8 P.M.–10 A.M.)

- 10 a.m.: Breakfast – French toast with whole-grain bread, maple syrup, and berries
- 1 p.m.: Lunch – Massaged kale salad with crispy chickpeas
- 7 p.m.: Dinner – Tuna poké bowl

SUNDAY (FAST 8 P.M.–NOON)

- 10 a.m.: Breakfast – Two pasture-raised eggs over avocado toast with fruit
- 1 p.m.: Lunch – Tofu and vegetable rice bowl
- 7 p.m.: Dinner – Carne asada tacos

20-Hour Fast Every Day (a.k.a. Warrior)

The final variation of daily fasting is the 20/4, or Warrior, method. This style regulates eating to a four-hour window, while fasting the remaining 20 hours. It's modeled after how we believe our ancient ancestors ate. The Warrior method differs from the other methods in that it allows for very limited caloric intake during the fasting window, such as a splash of milk in your coffee or savoring a hard-boiled egg. Essentially, it involves eating very little along with one balanced meal. This distinction makes it more approachable. The Warrior method can be implemented as part of a 12/14/16 TRF schedule by adding days of more restricted feeding windows. This can also be a good way to ease yourself into a weekly fasting routine by eating traditionally some days and choosing one or several days a week to implement this 20/4 fast.

Those who succeed using the Warrior method enjoy only dealing with one meal a day and report calming physiological responses and increased mental focus. Benefits stem from the stimulation of acute stress or the fight-or-flight response, which heightens the body's responses, boosting energy, cellular turnover, and alertness. A controlled trial of healthy, normal-weight adults showed that one meal a day (even without an overall calorie deficit) can stimulate modest changes in improved body composition and reduced cardiovascular risk. Due to the extended fasting period, you might expect to feel additional hunger, irritability, fatigue, headaches, or feeling full more quickly. This method is designed for women who already have fasting experience and should not be the first style of fasting you try, as it can disrupt hormones and lead to hypoglycemia. Be careful to not snack excessively throughout the fasting window. Those calories can easily add up and negate the benefits of this method. When it comes to your one meal, focus on lots of vegetables, a source of protein, and complex carbohydrates. Avoid processed foods, which can disturb digestion and hunger cues. It is up to you to choose which meal works the best for you. Many people with families or social commitments might want to keep dinner as their main meal, while those who start their day very early or conduct lunch meetings might want to prioritize their midday meal. If sustaining this style long term, a daily vitamin and electrolytes are advised.

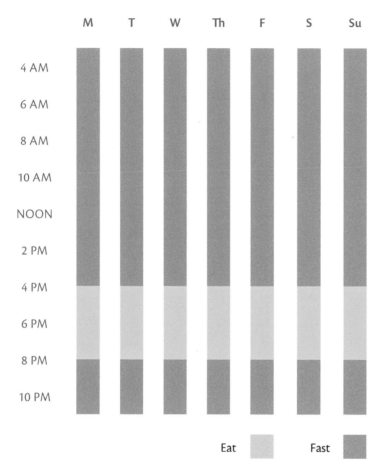

	M	T	W	Th	F	S	Su

4 AM

6 AM

8 AM

10 AM

NOON

2 PM

4 PM

6 PM

8 PM

10 PM

Eat   Fast

20-Hour Fast Meal Plan

This sample plan is for a full seven days of a Warrior-style fast—20 hours fasting and a four-hour eating window, prioritizing the dinner meal. While the example is for a full week, this style can be very effective and more sustainable if adopted only a couple days a week, especially at first.

MONDAY

- 4 p.m.: Snack – Two hard-boiled eggs, cut vegetables and hummus, and green tea
- 7 p.m.: Dinner – Fresh pasta with pesto, shredded kale salad, and a glass of wine

TUESDAY

- 4 p.m.: Snack – Endurance Indulgence (see page 72)
- 7 p.m.: Dinner – Herb-roasted free-range chicken with vegetables and potatoes

WEDNESDAY

- 4 p.m.: Snack – Two hard-boiled eggs, cut vegetables and hummus, and green tea
- 7 p.m.: Dinner – Margherita pizza with balsamic arugula salad

THURSDAY

- 4 p.m.: Snack – Kale and papaya smoothie with protein
- 7 p.m.: Dinner – Grass-fed flank steak with green beans and mushrooms, and a chunk of whole-grain sourdough bread with ghee

- 4 p.m.: Snack – Avocado toast and matcha tea
- 7 p.m.: Dinner – Sushi, seaweed salad, and sake

- 4 p.m.: Snack – Greek yogurt and cut fruit
- 7 p.m.: Dinner – Tandoori free-range chicken burger with sweet potato fries and tzatziki cucumbers

- 4 p.m.: Snack – Scrambled, pasture-raised eggs with fresh salsa
- 7 p.m.: Dinner – Tofu, buckwheat, and veggie bowl with spicy peanut sauce

WEEKLY FASTING PLANS

If the thought of following a fasting protocol each and every day seems overwhelming, you have the option of weekly fasting. Styles such as the 5:2 and alternate-day fasting are examples of weekly fasts. Fasting this way provides just as many benefits as TRF or daily fasting. You are likely to experience decreased bloating, improved mental focus, stabilized blood glucose levels, and reduced hunger even on non-fasting days. This method of fasting might be your best bet because it has been reported that caloric consumption naturally decreases by 20 percent following a fasting day. Full, 24-hour fasts might also work to better stimulate anti-aging and mental focus than other fasting protocols.

Weekly fasting has a slightly different protocol than other styles. Unlike daily fasted periods where all calories are avoided, 24-hour fasts limit caloric intake to less than 25 percent of your daily needs. This translates roughly to 500 calories for those normally consuming 2,000 calories a day. Using a food tracking app is helpful on fasting days to make sure you are not going over your allowed calories. Start slowly and ease into weekly, intermittent fasting styles. Health benefits can be seen from just one fasting day a week, so do not feel pressured to do more than your body can tolerate. While you'll be focusing less on when to eat and not eat, there are potential drawbacks to this style of intermittent fasting include fatigue, hunger, and headaches on the fasting day. To lessen any side effects, fill your day with light busy work and try to improve anti-stress self-care rituals, such as meditation, a nap, yoga, reading, being creative, or taking an outdoor stroll on your fasting day.

The 5:2 Fast

The most popular form of weekly fasting is the 5:2 method. This refers to fasting for two days a week, either back-to-back or nonconsecutively, with five days of regular eating. This can be a low-stress method because instead of worrying about what to eat for a week on a normal eating schedule or eating according to a time-restricted eating plan, you are only restricted two days a week. This style allows for a small amount, up to 25 percent, of calories to be consumed on the two fasting days, and the rest of the week resumes your normal healthy eating.

Due to this simple fasting design, it is one of the most well-studied styles of intermittent fasting. A 2010 study found that this form of fasting can provide women with the same weight loss benefits men enjoy. According to a 2018 study, placing the two fasting days together was shown to improve HbA1c, a measure of insulin resistance.

While two days of fasting are easier than seven, it is still difficult for your body to adjust to consuming a fraction of needed calories on those days. Pay attention to your body; some fatigue and brain fog are standard at first, but should dissipate as your body adjusts. Drinking plenty of water and tea on fasting days can help reduce the urge to eat. Try not to be overly active on these days; focus on leisurely walks or low-intensity exercises such as yoga to take your mind off food.

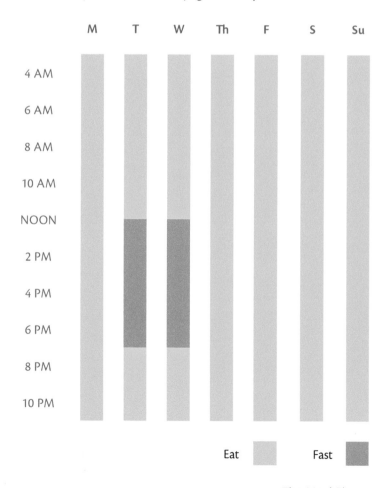

MONDAY

Consume a balanced, healthful diet.

TUESDAY (FASTING)

- Noon – Warm, organic Basic Bone Broth (see page 65)
- 4 p.m. – Ten steamed shrimp with two cups of shredded vegetables with vinegar and spices
- 7 p.m. – Unsweetened almond milk with protein powder

WEDNESDAY (FASTING)

- Noon – Warm water with lemon, steamed broccoli and two eggs
- 4 p.m. – Smoothie made with water, kale, ½ cup blueberries, 1 teaspoon coconut oil, and one scoop protein powder
- 7 p.m. – Two cups of Bone Broth-Based Miso Soup (see page 66) with tofu and spring onions

THURSDAY

Consume a balanced, healthful diet.

Consume a balanced, healthful diet.

Consume a balanced, healthful diet.

Consume a balanced, healthful diet.

Alternate-Day Fasting

Alternate-day fasting (ADF) is a step up from the 5:2 style because it adds an additional fasting day. One day is spent fasting and the next is not, and then this on/off schedule repeats. This style is great for those looking for a streamlined experience. On fasting days, you can eat up to 25 percent of your needs; on non-fasting days, you basically eat what you want. One clinical trial evaluated participants using alternate-day fasting who consumed up to 125 percent of their caloric needs on non-fasting days and found that they still benefited. This format can be a good starting point for those who are currently obese and have struggled in the past with traditional calorie restriction methods. An animal study suggested there is evidence that ADF can improve insulin sensitivity and reduce chronic disease risk, yet this style of intermittent fasting has not been well studied in humans. However, one small study of three men found ADF to be a convincing therapeutic diet for the treatment of diabetes. The largest concern with this style of fasting is that a relatively large chunk of time is spent fasting, leading to low adherence. Spending every other day not eating a balanced diet also makes it difficult to get all the nutrients needed for good health without closely monitoring intake. For this reason, ADF should be used as a short-term tool to regain control of food intake, then transitioned into a style of eating that better promotes long-term health.

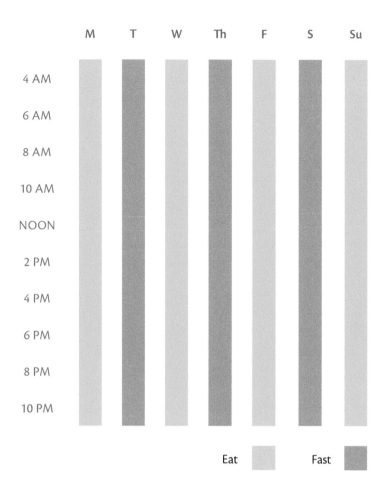

MONDAY

Consume a balanced, healthful diet.

TUESDAY (FASTING)

- Noon – Warm, organic Basic Bone Broth (page 65) and two cups of shredded vegetables with vinegar and spices
- 4 p.m. – Two ounces of gravlax with one apple
- 7 p.m. – Two cups of Bone Broth-Based Miso Soup (see page 66) with tofu and spring onions

WEDNESDAY

Consume a balanced, healthful diet.

THURSDAY (FASTING)

- Noon – Steamed, salted broccoli and Basic Bone Broth
- 4 p.m. – One cup of steamed edamame with lemon water
- 7 p.m. – Unsweetened almond milk blended with kale and protein powder

FRIDAY

Consume a balanced, healthful diet.

SATURDAY (FASTING)

- Noon – Warm water with lemon, steamed broccoli, and two eggs
- 4 p.m. – Smoothie made with water, kale, ½ cup blueberries, 1 teaspoon coconut oil, and one scoop protein powder
- 7 p.m. – One cup of Bone Broth-Based Miso Soup with tofu and spring onions

SUNDAY

Consume a balanced, healthful diet.

EXTENDED FASTS TO BE SCHEDULED MONTHLY OR YEARLY

Extended fasting is any protocol that takes your fast beyond 48 hours, such as a three-day fast or weeklong fast, and is only used monthly or annually as a type of reboot or system cleanse.

24- to 72-Hour Fasting

These fasts are popular among people looking to boost mental stimulation, promote anti-aging, reduce chronic stress, limit mental decline, and cleanse the body of excess toxins or junk that can build up throughout the year. Improved muscle tone will likely occur as well as weight loss; however, it will be temporary from water loss and will return once normal eating resumes. These extended fasts are difficult and only those who are in a relatively healthy state should attempt them. When fasting for days, expect to need a large amount of will-power, because experiencing extreme hunger is possible (although it might subside further into the fast). Headaches, dizziness, fatigue, shaking, low blood sugar, and low vitamin/mineral levels are all very possible and potentially dangerous side effects. Women who are currently experiencing hormonal imbalances, working toward fertility, or in very high-stress situations on a daily basis should not try this kind of fast, especially without the care of a health and nutrition expert. Before beginning a fast, ease into it with light but highly nutritious meals the day before. On fasting days, eat less than 25 percent of your caloric needs with plenty of electrolyte water to prevent dehydration. After fasting, return to normal eating but ease the body out of the fast with small, more frequent protein-packed meals.

Week 1

Consume a balanced, healthful diet.

Week 2

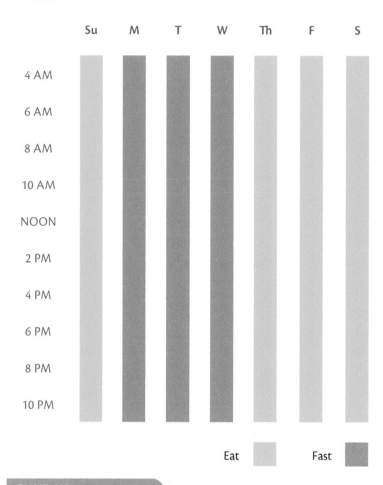

	Su	M	T	W	Th	F	S
4 AM							
6 AM							
8 AM							
10 AM							
NOON							
2 PM							
4 PM							
6 PM							
8 PM							
10 PM							

Eat   Fast

SUNDAY

Consume lighter meals today.

- Breakfast – Two eggs, smoked salmon, avocado, whole-grain toast, and a grapefruit
- Lunch – Grilled free-range chicken over shredded kale, blueberries, pecans, and tahini dressing
- Dinner – Tomato soup with roasted vegetables and toast with ghee

MONDAY (FASTING)

Abstain from food completely, or take in less than 25% of calories.

- Breakfast – Skip
- Lunch – Basic Bone Broth (see page 65)
- Dinner – Two hard-boiled eggs with sliced tomato

TUESDAY (FASTING)

- Breakfast – Morning Jump Start (see page 69)
- Lunch – Spaghetti squash with ghee
- Dinner – Basic Bone Broth

WEDNESDAY (FASTING)

- Breakfast – Skip
- Lunch – Bone Broth-Based Miso Soup (see page 66)
- Dinner – Skip

Ease back into eating with small, protein-rich meals.

- Breakfast – Two pasture-raised eggs with berries and coconut yogurt
- Snack – Fresh green juice
- Lunch – Wild salmon over soba noodles in miso broth and roasted broccoli
- Dinner – Baked tofu with butternut squash, buckwheat, tomatoes, green beans, and pesto

Consume a balanced, healthful diet.

Consume a balanced, healthful diet.

Week 3

Consume a balanced, healthful diet each day of the week.

Week 4

Consume a balanced, healthful diet each day of the week.

BREAKING YOUR FAST

Even if you had a wonderful fasting experience, returning to normal eating is the light at the end of the tunnel. Fasting is not meant to starve you, and returning to a good, healthful diet is what makes intermittent fasting sustainable and healthy. How you break the fast is an important part of the process, as being overly excited to resume eating can lead to eating too much too quickly and experiencing a rebound effect of cravings, gastric distress, and fatigue. The best thing you can do is plan your post-fast meal before you begin the fast. This will give you something to look forward to, provide consistency, and help ease your body into resuming digestion and calorie processing again. Start with a small meal that has more protein and fat with some complex carbohydrates. My favorite fast-breaking meal is eggs with sweet potato and vegetable hash cooked with avocado. If you feel too full, too bloated, or otherwise too sensitive to eat a full meal after fasting, I advise using the Mental Joe or Endurance Indulgence recipes listed in chapter 4 to ease your way from fasting to consuming calories again. Avoiding simple sugars in your first meal will help keep blood glucose levels stable. Always listen to your body and learn to be intuitive about giving it what it needs.

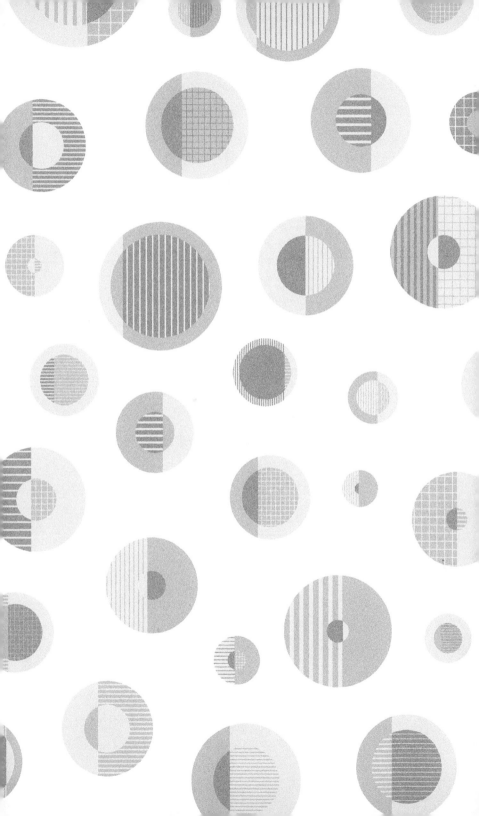

CHAPTER FOUR

Tools and Tips for Your Fast

Your fast should be enjoyable and have a positive impact on your health and lifestyle. Let's review a few important factors that can contribute to a successful fasting experience, including recipes and best practices.

WHAT TO DRINK

Liquids are an important part of fasting as they provide vital hydration and can provide nutrients during your fast. Here are a few liquids that can make your fast a more healthful experience.

Bone Broths

Bone broth is made by simmering the connective tissue and bones of an animal in water with vegetables, spices, and herbs. The end result is an almost meaty-tasting broth that is very satisfying to sip. When fasts allow low-calorie intake, sipping bone broth is a way to settle an empty stomach without breaking your fast. During regular food intake, broths can enhance meals by replacing liquids used to cook rice, quinoa, and sauces. These broths also offer a plethora of nutrients that help keep a body healthy, such as iron, amino acids, calcium, magnesium, zinc, and selenium. Numerous potential health benefits include improved joint health, mental clarity, reduced hunger, improved sleep, and better digestion. To get a variety of vitamins and minerals, make batches from different animal sources, like chicken, turkey, fish, and cattle. Using free-range, organic, and local ingredients is important for getting the best profile of fatty acids and nutrients.

There are several nutritious brands of bone broth available in grocery stores. Look for them in shelf-stable containers by the other soups, refrigerated near kombucha-style beverages, and in the freezer section. Making bone broths at home is a simple culinary adventure that can let you customize flavors.

Non-bone broths, including vegetable broths, can still be a great way to flavor your meals but won't offer the same health properties. Bouillon cubes and other highly processed products should be avoided.

BASIC BONE BROTH

Serves 5 | Prep time: 20 minutes | Cook time: 9 hours

While store brands are accessible and easy, making your own bone broth is a simple way to fit a broth to your personal taste, use up leftover scraps, and always have broth on hand. I love making batches throughout the year, using up seasonal scraps of herbs and vegetable bits lingering in my fridge along with bones obtained from a local butcher. This basic, strained bone broth is suitable for alternate-day fasting and extended fasts. You can also use it during fed periods as a base to rice or stews.

2–4 pounds animal parts (bone, marrow, connective tissue, etc.)
2 carrots, peeled and chopped
2–4 celery stalks, chopped
1 tablespoon olive oil
1 gallon water
2 tablespoons apple cider vinegar
1 onion, peeled and diced
2 garlic cloves, finely chopped
Flavor to taste: Try salt, pepper, herbs, chilies, aminos,
     miso, seaweed

1. Preheat the oven to 450°F.

2. Roast the bones, carrots, and celery in the oil for about 30 minutes, tossing the ingredients halfway through.

3. Remove from the oven and add the water, vinegar, onion, and garlic to a large pot, over medium-high heat, and bring to a boil. Flavor to taste.

4. Reduce to a simmer and cover for at least 8 hours. Cooking longer, up to a full day, allows more nutrients to seep into the broth.

5. Strain, saving the broth and discarding the solids.

6. Consume immediately or batch into small containers and refrigerate. Try adding the liquid to ice cube molds and freezing for later.

Per Serving: Calories: 40; Total fat: 0g; Total carbohydrates: 0g; Net carbs: 0g;
Fiber: 0g; Protein: 10g

BONE BROTH-BASED MISO SOUP

Serves 2–4 | Prep time: 10 minutes | Cook time: 15 minutes

This is a personal favorite of mine as I find the taste of miso to be incredibly earthy and savory. It also fills the house with a wonderful aroma. This soup is appropriate for extended fasts when very small amounts of calories are allowed. It can easily be made into a full, balanced meal for non-fasting periods by adding brown rice or soba. This broth is loaded with healing, balancing, and immunity-boosting benefits.

2 cups Basic Bone Broth (see page 65)
2 cups water
1 tablespoon nori
2–4 tablespoons miso paste, depending on taste
4 scallions, sliced
1 cup sliced shiitake mushrooms
½ (14-ounce block) firm tofu, cubed
1 tablespoon aminos

1. Combine the bone broth, water, nori, miso, scallions, mushrooms, tofu, and aminos in a large pot over medium heat and bring to a simmer.

2. Simmer until the miso paste is dissolved into the liquid.

3. Ladle into bowls and serve.

Per Serving: Calories: 109; Total fat: 3g; Total carbohydrates: 6g; Net carbs: 4g; Fiber: 2g; Protein: 10g

Coffee

Coffee provides an energy and alertness boost along with several health benefits related to its antioxidant and flavonol content. It also increases fat burning, making it an ideal accompaniment to your fast. During 12- to 16-hour fasts, stick with black coffee because adding anything will break the fast. For 20- or 24-hour fasts, adding a few calories to your cup can help provide enough satiety to manage the fasting hours without disrupting your metabolic system. When your fast is finished, you may include coffee and coffee beverages as part of your regular nutrition plan.

If your fasting goals include hormone balance and mood stabilization, coffee might be a triggering item for you. Women tend to metabolize caffeine slowly, leading to increased anxiety and poor sleep. In this circumstance, slowly and consistently reduce the amount of caffeine you take in; your body is sensitive to change. Adding decaf varieties is a nice way to get health benefits without the jitters. Pay attention to how your body reacts to caffeine's stimulatory effects and sip accordingly.

Additions such as milk, fats, sweeteners, and extras can impact your coffee's healthfulness, so choose wisely. Milks can be a way to boost creaminess and mellow bitter coffee. Any milk is fine as long as it works well for your body and overall diet. Unsweetened nut milks can be low in calories, making them ideal for fasting hours. A splash of grass-fed cow's or goat's milk can provide omega fatty acids, calcium, and vita-min D. If you find dairy hard to digest or irritating to your skin or mood, stick with a plant-based source. Oat and pea milk are nut-free, plant-based options. Soy milk should be avoided as there is potential for excessive soy intake disrupting female hormones. Adding clarified butter, coconut oil, or even nut butters boost the fat profile of your coffee, creating a slow-digesting response to boost satiety, limit cravings, and enhance mental concentration. This can be very helpful to your fast. Sweeteners come in many forms: honey, maple syrup, table sugar, coconut sugar, corn syrup, etc. Adding these to black coffee is not advised because it promotes insulin spikes, which leads to a roller coaster of energy levels and cravings. Adding a small amount of a sweetener containing fat to your coffee is less damaging as the fat blunts the quick absorption of the sugar.

There are many extras that can give your beverage and health an added boost. These include—but aren't limited to—rishi, ginger, cordyceps, collagen powders, cayenne, cinnamon, cacao, and maca. I suggest purchasing a milk-frothing wand to better blend in your coffee additions.

MORNING JUMP START

Serves 1 | Prep time: 2 minutes

This simple coffee variation is my go-to for kick-starting a busy day while fasting. The cayenne adds a metabolic boost and ginger calms the stomach. It is appropriate for drinking during your fasts.

Pinch cayenne
Pinch cinnamon
Pinch ginger
1 cup coffee

Mix the cayenne, cinnamon, and ginger into the coffee and sip. Can be served hot or iced.

Per Serving: Calories: 4; Total fat: 0g; Total carbohydrates: 0.5g; Net carbs: 0.2g; Fiber: 0.3g; Protein: 0g

MENTAL JOE

Serves 1 | Prep time: 2 minutes

I rely on this option when I have a busy workday and need extreme mental focus as rishi, a mushroom extract, can improve irritability and fatigue. This drink is appropriate for extended fasting periods or breaking a fast and preparing the body for a full meal.

1 teaspoon rishi, a powdered mushroom supplement available at most health food stores or online

½ teaspoon ghee

½ teaspoon coconut oil

1 cup coffee

Stir the rishi, ghee, and coconut oil into the coffee until dissolved. Enjoy.

KITCHEN TIP: A milk-frothing wand works well for mixing these drinks.

Per Serving: Calories: 44; Total fat: 5g; Total carbohydrates: 0g; Net carbs: 0g; Fiber: 0g; Protein: 0g

CHILLED MIDDAY BOOST

Serves 1 | Prep time: 2 minutes

I frequently sip this as a late morning pick-me-up on a hot day. It is appropriate for extended fasts or non-fasting periods.

½ cup tonic
½ orange, juiced
2 shots espresso, cooled

Combine the tonic and juice of the orange into the espresso and serve.

Per Serving: Calories: 62; Total fat: 0g; Total carbohydrates: 15g; Net carbs: 15g; Fiber: 0g; Protein: 0g

ENDURANCE INDULGENCE

Serves 1 | Prep time: 5 minutes

This is more smoothie than coffee! After a fasted workout, this is my go-to for promoting energy, collagen repair, and satiety. It can also be used as a meal replacement or to break a fasting period without straining the gut.

1 cup coffee or 2 espresso shots, cooled
1 cup milk of choice
1 tablespoon cashew butter
1 tablespoon maple syrup
1 scoop collagen powder
1 teaspoon maca
Pinch cinnamon
Pinch salt

Combine the coffee or espresso, milk, cashew butter, maple syrup, collagen powder, maca, cinnamon, and salt in a blender and blend until smooth.

Per Serving: Calories: 320; Total fat: 13g; Total carbohydrates: 31g; Net carbs: 29g; Fiber: 2g; Protein: 22g

Tea

Fresh-brewed, plain tea offers a large variety of health-boosting benefits and is often used to sooth ailments and calm the body. Just like coffee, be mindful of the caffeine content and that what you choose to add to your tea can affect your fast and health in different ways. Pay attention to how your body feels after drinking different tea varieties and adjust consumption accordingly.

Other Liquids

While water should be your main source of hydration at all times, there are other beverages you can drink. During your fast, choose very low or zero-calorie beverages. When including beverages as caloric options, look for those that use whole ingredients with no added sugars; they can be a hydrating source of nutrients but many are loaded with sugar and calories. It is important to note that beverages can taste very sweet without added sugar. For instance, some whole ingredients, such as carrots and apples, taste very sweet after being juiced. Aim to stay away from sugar-free alternatives (including Stevia, erythritol, and so on) because they can disrupt your body's natural responses to sugar and calories. Aim to sip your beverages slowly, and do not regularly replace meals with drinks because your body does not experience the same signals of fullness when the chewing process is bypassed. The following recipes are my go-to options for juices and elixirs to boost my mood, energy, and metabolism.

HERBACEOUS REFRESHER

Makes about 3 (3-ounce) servings* | Prep time: 10 minutes

This juice will hydrate, freshen, and energize your body while providing concentrated phytonutrients. I make this blend every couple of days and sip it first thing in the morning to recharge my system. I might also drink a couple of ounces on days my vegetable intake is limited. I suggest you drink 2 to 4 ounces, topped with sparkling water.

1 head organic romaine lettuce
2 celery stalks
1 large cucumber
1 green pepper
1 small bunch of parsley, trimmed
½ lemon, peeled, seeded
1-inch chunk peeled ginger

1. Combine the lettuce, celery, cucumber, pepper, parsley, lemon, and ginger into a blender or juicer, and blend until smooth (if using a blender, strain if desired).

2. Consume immediately or refrigerate in a sealed container for up to 2 days.

Per Serving (assuming 3 cups liquid): Calories: 13; Total fat: 0g; Total carbohydrates: 3g; Net carbs: 2g; Fiber: 1g; Protein: 1g

*Volume will vary based on water content of vegetables.

JUST-SPICY-ENOUGH CITRUS ENERGIZER

Serves 1 | Prep time: 5 minutes

Interesting fact: Just the smell of grapefruit can boost your mental energy and stimulate weight loss. I often pair this beverage with my first meal of the day to enhance metabolic action.

1 grapefruit
8 ounces alkaline water
1 tablespoon honey or maple syrup (optional)
Pinch cayenne

1. Juice the grapefruit, add water as desired.

2. Mix in honey or syrup and cayenne.

Per Serving: Calories: 76; Total fat: 0g; Total carbohydrates: 18g; Net carbs: 18g; Fiber: 0g; Protein: 1g

MORINGA PERSON

If you are avoiding coffee or simply looking to improve nutrient consumption, this drink is loaded with antioxidants and provides a calming effect. Moringa is a green plant powder supplement with a grassy, earthy flavor almost like matcha. Sip this on your extended fasts or use it to ease out of a fast before consuming solid food again.

1 tablespoon moringa powder
1 cup unsweetened almond milk
½ tablespoon coconut oil
1 tablespoon honey

On the stove, gently heat and stir together the moringa powder, milk, coconut oil, and honey until warm and well mixed.

Per Serving: Calories: 172; Total fat: 9g; Total carbohydrates: 23g; Net carbs: 21g; Fiber: 2g; Protein: 2g

TIPS AND BEST PRACTICES

Tackling a new process is bound to come with a few challenges. Feeling confident with your choice to fast is key, but it is also very helpful to prepare for situations and issues that might arise.

Drink Lots of Water

Drink water! Yes, this has been mentioned before, but it is crucial to maintaining hydration, limiting hunger, and improving digestion during your fasting periods. How much you should drink depends on your body size, the climate where you live, and how much you sweat. In general, sip throughout the day. Adding a pinch of salt or an electrolyte tablet to water helps maintain essential mineral content while fasting.

Use Calorie Counters

Counting calories and tracking food intake can be a total chore. It can also be a very useful tool when trying to adhere to a plan and make dietary changes. Track your intake occasionally just to check in and be aware of what you are eating. When adjusting to consuming less than 25 percent of your caloric needs on full-day or extended fasts, counting calories is a must. There are many free apps, such as CalorieKing or MyFitnessPal, that allow you to easily keep track. Once you have a grasp on what 25 percent of your intake looks like, you can stop counting. This process is meant to help you manage your fast, not put additional stress or restraints on your life and nutrition.

Don't Rearrange Social Plans

A large part of your fasting success depends on your ability to maintain consistency and confidence throughout your journey. Living your life as you normally would is the best way to do this. Aim to maintain a normal schedule, including social events and meetups. See the sidebar for help navigating social situations.

No Need to Tell Others Unless It Comes Up

Disclosing your fast is a personal choice. There is no need to announce your lifestyle habits to anyone if you aren't comfortable doing so. Telling others you are fasting could result in a bombardment of questions and possible judgment. If you enjoy having that discussion with others, great! For those who don't want to defend or explain their choices to family, friends, or strangers, simply sidestep the issue.

Quieting Stomach Growls

Physically and mentally, we become very accustomed to routine and consistency. Most of us eat at the same times each day, and making big shifts in this can cause the body to signal that something is off. When you skip a meal, your body might respond with a grumbling stomach. Have a cup of water or tea, do some busy work, or take a short walk. The grumbling will likely subside because the pains are temporary and will lessen as your body adjusts to your fasting schedule and expects food at different times.

Other Practical Concerns

Flexibility: Thinking about scheduling eating/not eating for your day, week, or month can be a bit overwhelming. While it requires a bit of structure and consistency, there is a great deal of flexibility. If you have a stressful work presentation coming up, are off on an exciting vacation, or simply need a break from the schedule, it is absolutely fine to skip the upcoming fast and resume with the next one. Occasionally missing a fast or even fasting only occasionally can still provide health benefits.

Exercise: Exercising is crucial to a healthy, well-functioning body. Physical exercise of all types and intensities can fit into your life, even when committed to a fasting routine. Replace intense or high-duration workouts with short, light exercises on days you abstain from food. Simply pay attention to your body and energy levels and pull back when your body needs rest.

Eat nutritiously: Fasting is the easy part of this lifestyle plan. Even when you're not fasting, choosing healthful food can still cause some confusion. Fill your plate mostly with unprocessed, colorful food ingredients, enjoy the occasional indulgence, and stay away from overly restrictive fad diets. Focus on behaviors associated with eating, such as being aware of hunger cues, chewing thoroughly, eating slowly, being mindful of food consumption, and paying attention to your body's unique needs, as these are just as vital as good nutrition.

Plateaus: Plateaus in health and weight happen when our actions become stagnant or we have progressed to a point beyond what our original behavioral changes can support. This is often a frustrating point to reach; however, it is a normal part of progressing to our ultimate goals. When you hit a plateau that lasts several weeks, it is time to shake up your routine. The easiest way to jump-start your body's response is by switching fasting methods. For example, if you were doing the Crescendo method, switch to the 5:2 to shake things up. Beyond your fasting regimen, it might be time to focus more on food choices and exercise habits to meet your ultimate goal(s).

HOW TO NAVIGATE SOCIAL SITUATIONS WHILE FASTING

Fasting can be awkward during social situations that revolve around food. Staying committed to your health-improving goals is more important than eating something out of obligation. If you are questioned about not eating and don't want to share that you're fasting, provide a simple and definitive answer, such as "not hungry," "suffering indigestion," or that you just ate. Holding a cup of water, tea, or coffee is a good way to not look empty-handed and avoid food and drink offers. Take this opportunity to enjoy other aspects of being around people, such as engaging in deep conversation (you can't really do that with your mouth full). For the most part, you can schedule fasting times around social events you would like to eat at. Of course, you can take part in and thoroughly enjoy any social event without consuming food and drink. For those events that just would not be meaningful to you without raising a toast or enjoying a bite, simply fast on another day or timeline.

FREQUENTLY ASKED QUESTIONS (FAQS)

To help ease your anxiety about starting a fasting regimen, let's discuss some frequently asked questions.

How should I handle alcohol consumption while fasting?

Moderate alcohol consumption for women is defined as one serving per day and can be safe and even healthful. When fasting, remember that the effects of alcohol will be felt faster and stronger on an empty stomach. Consuming alcohol is not suggested during fasting periods for this reason. You'll also want to limit alcohol before beginning a fasting period.

Can I put powdered vitamin supplements like Airborne/Emergen-C® in my water?

You can absolutely utilize water supplements to boost nutrient levels during your fast. However, stay away from products with calories, sugars, and artificial ingredients.

Should I take a multivitamin daily while fasting?

Daily vitamins shouldn't be relied on to obtain all necessary vitamins and minerals, but they can be a great way to cover your bases, especially when fasting. Skip gummy vitamins because they typically contain sugar and calories.

Can I eat mints or chew gum during my fast?

Mints and gums should be avoided while fasting. Those that contain sugar and/or calories are not appropriate for fasting. Artificial ingredients in sugar-free options can destroy a healthy gut biome and lead to bloating. Chewing anything signals food intake to the brain and can mess up the signaling and hunger responses that fasting works to improve.

Can I eat/drink things with aspartame or other artificial sweeteners during my fast?

If consuming some sugar-free products during your fast helps you get started, then the good likely outweighs the negative. Ultimately, you'll want to forgo all artificial sweeteners because they can potentially trigger the insulin response, mess with hunger sensations, and reduce a healthy gut biome.

Why are fasting timeframes always listed in even numbers (12/14/16)? Can I do a 13-hour fast, for instance?

Even intervals are easier to structure for most people. The fasting benefits truly begin at 12 hours, so as long as your fast goes beyond that, 13 or 15 hours is just fine if that works best for your schedule.

Should I eat large meals when not fasting?

You should eat meal portions that your body needs. Eat slowly, chew thoroughly, and stop eating when you feel satisfied. There is no reason to eat extra-large portions to compensate for calories not consumed while fasting.

BEYOND FASTING

Fasting is a simple and unintimidating way to start improving your health because it doesn't necessarily involve changing your diet. However, to take advantage of this lifestyle change and make it as effective as possible, there are dietary improvements you can work toward.

Believe it or not, once you begin fasting, your body will crave and thrive on healthier food choices. Adding highly processed and heavy foods after a fast can cause gastric disturbances, digestive issues, and mood and energy swings. As you progress on your fasting journey, be aware of how your body responds to what you feed it and adjust accordingly. You might be surprised at how your food intake naturally changes simply as a response to the fast. Filling your plate with high-quality proteins, fiber-filled complex carbohydrates, satisfying fats, and nutrient-rich produce from natural sources will help you maximize health and weight results.

Eating LCHF or Keto

Many will want to experiment with eating a low-carb high-fat (LCHF) diet or ketogenic diet in addition to their fasting efforts. Ketogenic diets are thought to ease the transition in and out of fasting periods by keeping the body running on fat and maintaining stable blood glucose levels. Consuming a high proportion of calories from fat also helps one feel more satiated and better able to maintain a fasting regimen. LCHF diets are a less extreme version of the ketogenic diet, which relies on consuming a mere 5 to 10 percent of calories a day from carbohydrates. A single banana would meet the diet's carb cap.

If weight loss and/or diabetes is your main concern, some research supports that this style of eating can be beneficial. When carbohydrates are restricted almost completely, the body lacks an immediate energy source, and your metabolism is forced to tap into burning stored fat for fuel. However, women concerned with athletic performance, hormone balance, and fertility should not overly restrict carbohydrate intake. Instead, they should consume whole sources of carbohydrates such as sweet potatoes, fruit, and oats while limiting processed, refined sources such as candy, cereals, and packaged breads. While potentially promising, consuming a very imbalanced macronutrient distribution such as LCHF and keto is still considered experimental because the long-term health effects have not been extensively documented. Consult with a nutrition professional and your physician first.

TRUST YOUR BODY

Fasting is not a replacement for a healthy, nutrient-rich diet. It should be used as a tool to aid you in achieving your health goals. Intermittent fasting should be a positive experience. Throughout your process, check in on your reasons for starting the fast and how your body is responding to it. The most important thing anyone can do is be aware of choices and behaviors that affect health goals and constantly work to make improvements. Tune in, be mindful, and adjust your actions accordingly. Fasting is not a punishment for your body; it's just the opposite, really. It is a way to reset internally and restore your body and mind to a healthy place. If fasting doesn't work for you, do not force it. Your body is with you for life. Treat it with respect and admiration.

Resources

I always suggest having additional resources about a topic that concerns health and wellness. Here are a few of my favorite sources for increasing my knowledge.

The Complete Guide to Nutritional Health is a book that has sat on my shelf for many years. It is a go-to for looking up holistic uses of foods/nutrients.

Today's Dietitian (todaysdietitian.com) is a great website that consults educated, registered dietitians on science-backed topics regarding food, health, and wellness.

Dr. Will Bulsiewicz is a gastroenterologist well versed in the gut-health relationship. He is a great resource for balanced, sound nutrition advice (theplantfedgut.com).

MindBodyGreen (mindbodygreen.com) is a wellness website that provides a fun variety of topics, from the science-backed to more questionable, but still inspirational, trends.

Deepak Chopra, M.D. (chopra.com/bios/deepak-chopra) is a pioneer of integrative medicine and blending Eastern practices with Western medicine. I highly recommend exploring his work.

Hungry for Results (hungryforresults.com) is a dietitian's website focused on nutrition and fitness that also has many original recipes and tips on intermittent fasting.

Mini Habits for Weight Loss: Stop Dieting. Form New Habits. Change Your Lifestyle Without Suffering by Stephen Guise can help set small behavioral changes that lead to big lifestyle improvements.

Ruffage: A Practical Guide to Vegetables by Abra Berens is a wonderful cookbook that helps you learn to use seasonal produce in simple yet elevated ways and improves the nutrition of your food choices when not fasting.

Fast Diets for Dummies by Kellyann Petrucci and Patrick Flynn—if you're looking for a simplified version of fasting, the For Dummies series has you covered.

Headspace.com: Applying meditation practices is a wonderful way to ease the body into a place of mental calm and focus.

Fasting apps: Use technology to help you stick to your fasting times, track goals, and stay focused. The following are available on Android and iPhone: MyFast, BodyFast, and Vora.

References

Antoni, R., K.L. Johnston, A.L. Collins, and M.D. Robertson. "Investigation into the acute effects of total and partial energy restriction on postprandial metabolism among overweight/obese participants," *British Journal of Nutrition* 115, no. 6 (March 28, 2016): 951–9.

Arciero, P.J., M.I. Goran, and E.T. Poehiman. "Resting metabolic rate is lower in women than in men," *Journal of Applied Physiology* 75, no. 6 (December 1993): 2514–20.

Barnosky, A.R., K.K. Hoddy, T.G. Unterman, and K.A. Varady. "Intermittent fasting vs daily calorie restriction for type 2 diabetes prevention: a review of human findings," *Translational Research* 164, no. 4 (October 2014): 302–11.

Carter, S., P.M. Clifton, and J.B. Keogh. "Effect of Intermittent Compared with Continuous Energy Restricted Diet on Glycemic Control in Patients with Type 2 Diabetes: A Randomized Noninferiority Trial," *JAMA Network Open* 1, no. 3 (July 20, 2018): e180756.

Centers for Disease Control and Prevention. "Folic Acid." Accessed September 2019. https://www.cdc.gov/ncbddd/folicacid/features/folic-acid.html.

Coller, R. "Intermittent fasting: the science of going without," *Canadian Medical Association Journal* 185, no. 9 (June 2013): E363–E364.

Cribbet, M.R., R.W. Logan, M.D. Edwards, E. Hanlon, C. Peek, J.J. Stubblefield, et al. "Circadian rhythms and metabolism: from the brain to the gut and back again," *Annals of the New York Academy of Sciences* 1385, no. 1 (December 2016): 21–40.

De Baaij, J.G., J.G. Hoenderop, and R.J. Bindels. "Magnesium in man: implications for health and disease," *Physiology Reviews* 95, no. 1 (January 2015): 1–46.

Engstrom, B.E., P. Burman, C. Holdstock, and F.A. Karlsson. "Effects of growth hormone (GH) on ghrelin, leptin, and adiponectin in

GH-deficient patients," *Journal of Clinical Endocrinology & Metabolism* 88, no. 11 (November 2003): 5193–8.

Furmli, S., R. Elmasry, M. Ramos, and J. Fung. "Therapeutic use of intermittent fasting for people with type 2 diabetes as an alternative to insulin," Case Reports 2018; 2018: bcr-2017-221854.

Gelino S., and M. Hansen. "Autophagy—An Emerging Anti-Aging Mechanism," *Journal of Clinical and Experimental Pathology* Suppl. 4 (July 12, 2012): 006.

Harvie, M.N., M. Pegington, M.P. Mattson, J. Frystyk, B. Dillon, G. Evans, et al. "The effects of intermittent or continuous energy restriction on weight loss and metabolic disease risk markers: a randomised trial in young overweight women," *International Journal of Obesity* 35, no. 5 (May 2011): 714–727.

Ho, K.Y., J.D. Veldhuis, M.L. Johnson, R. Furlanetto, W.S. Evans, K.G. Alberti, and M.O. Thorner. "Fasting enhances growth hormone secretion and amplifies the complex rhythms of growth hormone secretion in man," *Journal of Clinical Investigation* 81, no. 4 (April 1988): 968–975.

LeChaminant, J.D., E. Christenson, B.W. Baily, and L.A. Tucker. "Restricting night-time eating reduces daily energy intake in healthy young men: a short-term cross-over study," *British Journal of Nutrition* 110, no. 11 (December 14, 2013): 2108–13.

Longo, V.D., and S. Panda. "Fasting, circadian rhythms, and time restricted feeding in healthy lifespan," *Cell Metabolism* 23, no. 6 (June 14, 2016): 1048–1059.

MRC Vitamin Study Research Group. "Prevention of neural tube defects: Results of the Medical Research Council Vitamin Study," *The Lancet* 338, no. 8760 (July 1991): 131–137.

Rodríguez-Morán, M., and F. Guerroro-Romero. "Oral magnesium supplementation improves insulin sensitivity and metabolic control in type 2 diabetic subjects: a randomized double-blind controlled trial," *Diabetes Care* 26, no. 4 (April 2003): 1147–52.

Stote, K.S., D.J. Baer, K. Spears, D.R. Paul, G.K. Harris, W.V. Rumpler, et al. "A controlled trial of reduced meal frequency without caloric restriction in healthy, normal-weight, middle-aged adults," *The American Journal of Clinical Nutrition* 85, no. 4 (April 2007): 981–988.

Trepanowski, J.F., C.M. Kroeger, A. Barnosky, et al. "Effect of Alternate-Day Fasting on Weight Loss, Weight Maintenance, and Cardioprotection Among Metabolically Healthy Obese Adults: A Randomized Clinical Trial," *JAMA Internal Medicine* 177, no. 7 (2017): 930–938.

Varady, K.A., and M.K. Hellerstein. "Alternate-day fasting and chronic disease prevention: a review of human and animal trials," *The American Journal of Clinical Nutrition* 86, no. 1 (July 2007): 7–13.

Index

Acknowledgments

Living a healthy lifestyle takes support. It takes someone understanding that you simply must have kombucha in the fridge and sprouted brown rice on repeat order from Amazon, that the clock dictates eating on some days, and that the day might not be pleasant if a morning run is skipped. I am devoted to my lifestyle and I must thank my husband, Luke Russell, who not only tolerates but supports (and sometimes even participates in) these wellness practices.

About the Author

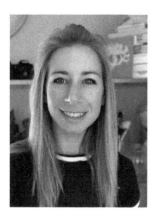

Lori Russell, MS, RD, CSSD, is a dietitian, wellness coach, personal trainer, recipe developer, athlete, and writer. She holds a master's degree in nutrition, is board certified as a sports specialist, and is currently completing her second master's in exercise science from Concordia University of St. Paul, Minnesota. Beyond traditional education, she has racked up twelve years of professional experience in the dynamic field of wellness, specializing in fueling performances, weight control, and whole-food nutrition. Being an elite road-cycling and distance-running athlete along with being diagnosed with celiac disease has contributed to her firsthand commitment to using wellness techniques to boost performance and health. Through her company Hungry for Results, Lori has worked with many food brands to develop recipes and content and has counseled individuals to improve their quality of life and athletic performance through behavior and food changes, and she writes nutrition content for many highly regarded publications. She is also the author of *The 30-Day Whole Food Meal Plan and Cookbook.*